Aqua Therapy for Lipedema and Lymphedema

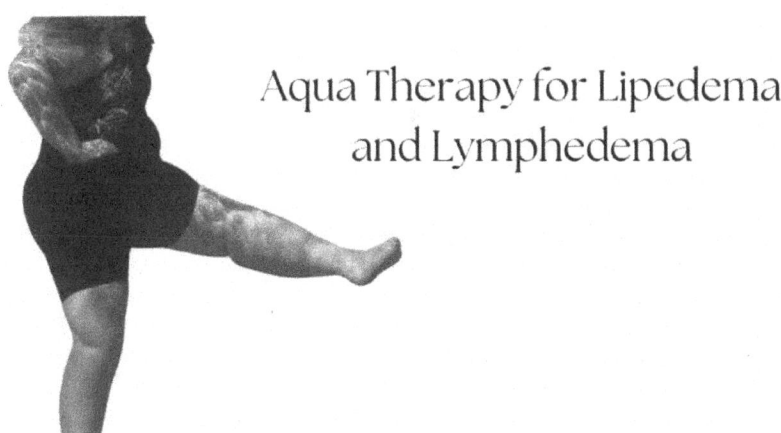

Aqua Therapy for Lipedema and Lymphedema

Aqua therapy for Lipedema and Lymphedema

The Gift of Water as Compression and for More Comfortable Physical Activity

(Black and White Edition)

Susan O'Hara

Foreword by LaNese Cummings, PT

Note to the Reader: This publication contains the opinions and ideas of its author(s). It is intended to provide helpful and informative material on the subject matter covered. It is sold with the understanding that the author(s) and publisher are not engaged in rendering professional services in the book. If the reader requires personal assistance or advice, a competent professional should be consulted. The author(s) and publisher specifically disclaim any responsibility for any liability, loss, or risk, personal or otherwise, which is incurred as a consequence, directly or indirectly, of the use and application of any of the contents of this book.

You are not alone! With millions of people in the world having lipedema and lymphedema, it's time to receive the care and products we need to live our best lives.

This book is available at a special discount when purchased in bulk for sales promotions, premiums, fund-raising, or educational use. For details, contact Susan O'Hara, LegsLikeMine@gmail.com with the subject: Bulk Sales.

Photography by Rob O'Hara. Styling by Morgan O'Hara.
Copyright 2023 Susan O'Hara. All rights reserved. No part of this work may be reproduced by any means, copied or distributed without express written permission of the author.
All rights reserved. Published 2023
www.LegsLikeMine.com

Library of Congress Cataloguing-in-Publication Data

Names: O'Hara, Susan, 1973-, author.
Title: Aqua therapy for Lipedema and Lymphedema: The Gift of Water as Compression and for More Comfortable Physical Activity (Black and White Edition) / Susan O'Hara
Description: Oklahoma City: 2023.
Includes bibliographical references.

Identifiers: ISBN: 9798387960505 (paperback)

Subjects: BISAC: HEALTH & FITNESS / Diseases / Lymphatics / Lipedema MEDICAL / Public Health | HEALTH & FITNESS / Women's Health / Mental Health

pIndependently published.

QR Codes Included

This book has the added feature of QR codes to get you where you want to be quickly, without having to type in long web addresses.

According to support.apple.com, to use a QR code from your Apple device:

1. Open the Camera app from your Home Screen, Control Center or Lock Screen.
2. Select the rear-facing camera. Hold your device so that the QR code appears in the viewfinder in the Camera app. Your device recognizes the QR code and shows a notification.
3. Tap the notification to open the link associated with the QR code.

QR Code Sample.

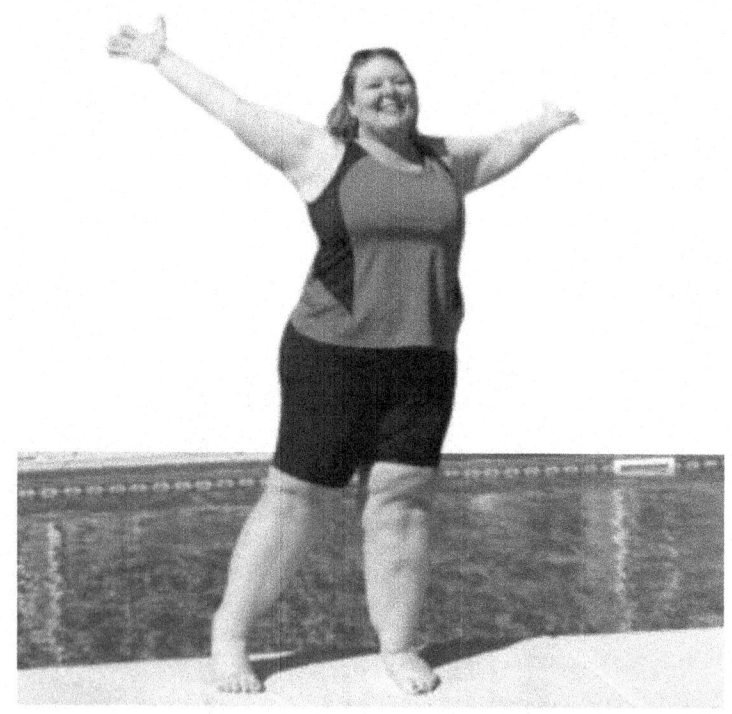

The author, modelling her lipedema-friendly swimsuit and feeling the joy of the water, at LegsLikeMine.com.

To my husband,

who goes along with whatever crazy idea I have and supports me however he is able, whether it's to stop and take pictures at my whim, give me unlimited IT help, put in a pool, review a book or support me in changing the focus of my life work.
Thank you for letting me be me.

With special thanks

To LaNese Cummings, my friend and Physical Therapist, and my caring friends in the physical and occupational therapy world,

and

To the online lipedema and lymphedema communities.

Aqua Therapy for Lipedema and Lymphedema

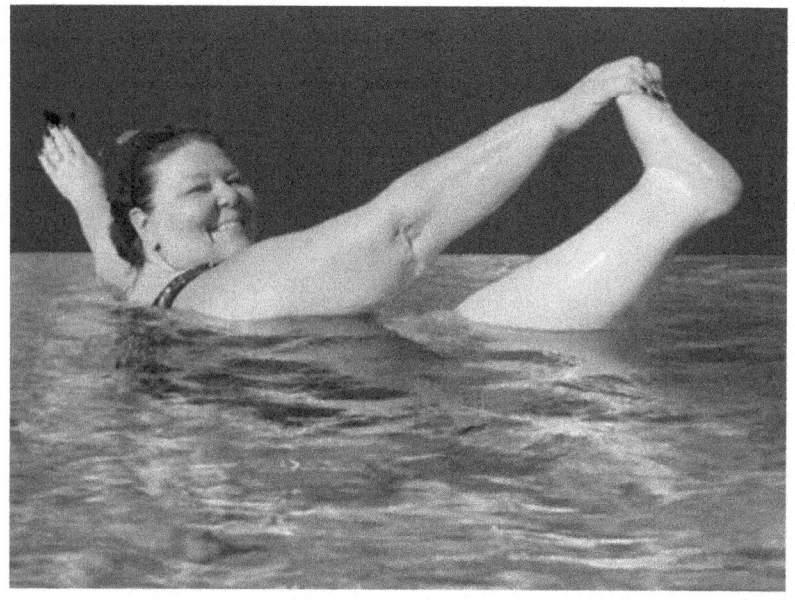

Being in the water gives me joy in being able to move in ways I would never try on land!

Contents

QR Codes Included	5
Foreword by LaNese Cummings, PT	13
About LaNese Cummings	14
Why Aqua therapy?	18
Water's Natural Compression	18
Swimming and Aqua therapy Are Good for our Mental Health!	19
Physical Benefits of Aqua therapy	20
Chapter 1: My Story	24
Chapter 2: What are Lipedema, Lymphedema and Fibrosis?	36
Lipedema	36
What Causes Lipedema?	43
Lymphedema	44
What Causes Lymphedema?	45
Fibrosis	46
Chapter 3: Water is Natural Compression	50
Why Compression is Important	50
How Water Compression Measures Up	50
How do Compression Garments Measure Up	51
Classes of Compression	51
Water Compression vs. Compression Garment Strength	52
Chapter 4: Aqua therapy Starts with the Mind	58
Affirmations	59
Sample Affirmations Related to Aqua therapy	61
Your Own Meaningful Affirmations	63
Progress, Not Perfection!	63

Chapter 5: Where and When to Swim	66
Where to Find "Your" Water	66
Could a Prescription for Swimming Help?	67
You Might Qualify for a Tax Deduction for an at-Home Pool	67
When to Swim	68
How Long to Swim in Each Session	68
How Often to Perform Aqua therapy	69
Chapter 6: Supplies	72
What to Wear	72
Confidence in a Swimming Suit	74
Caring for your Swimsuit	75
Other Supplies You Might Be Interested In	77
Chapter 7: Safety	82
Safety for Non-Swimmers	82
STOP! Contraindications for Aqua therapy	82
Fatigue	83
Water Temperature	84
Cleanliness	84
Hypermobility and Swimming	85
Don't Overdo It! And Other Random Safety Tips	88
Chapter 8: Aqua therapy Basics	92
General Tips on Exercising in the Water	93
Breathing	94
Simple Deep Abdominal Breathing	95
Take a Lymphatic Break!	96
Simple Abdominal Massage	96
Using Water Turbulence to Encourage Lymphatic Flow	98

Simple Self Leg Manual Lymphatic Drainage (MLD) in the Water	98
Basic Arm MLD in the Water	100
Put Your Compression Back On After Your Exercise, Every Time!	101
Modifying Exercises to Meet You Where You Are	101
Example Exercise Modifiers for Aquatic Moves	102
Chapter 9: Exercises	112
Cardio Exercises	113
Whole Body Exercises	118
Arm Exercises	119
Leg Exercises	128
Stretching Exercises	143
Pelvic Floor Exercises	159
How to do Kegel Exercises	159
Sample Workouts	160
Chapter 10: Resources and Support	166
Supply List with Links	168
Search Terms and Hashtags that might be helpful:	169
Behind the Scenes Fun	170
Bibliography	172
Aquatics	172
Lipedma	175
Lymphedema, Fibrosis and Oncology	176
Other Resources	178
Connect with LegsLikeMine	179

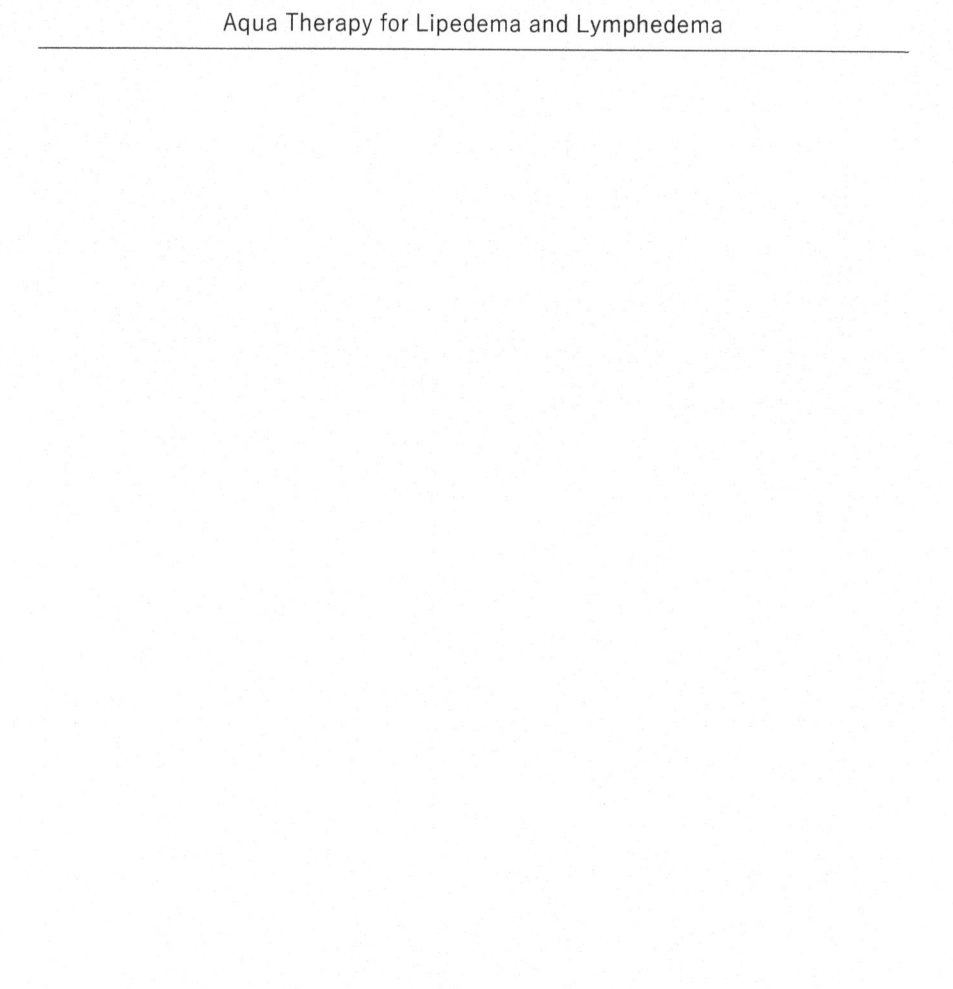

"I could float in the pool for hours, just letting the water carry me."

~ Jill Scott ~

Foreword
by LaNese Cummings, PT

Aquatic exercise is extremely beneficial for many different reasons! I encourage everyone to check with their doctors and determine if they are at a safe fitness level to participate in aqua therapy. Often, pain prevents many people from tolerating land-based workouts, but these same people can often thrive when utilizing aquatic exercise.

Being in water "unloads" the spine, which takes pressure off the discs, nerves, and joint surfaces. The unloading effect is like traction for the spine with up to 75% of the load removed from the spine when in chest-deep water. This unloading allows for improved freedom of motion and sends increased nutrients to the joints.

Our joints naturally do not have good blood flow, so for them to be healthy they need motion, which lubricates the joint. Therapists often say, "the motion is the lotion." Unfortunately, when we are in pain our brains tell us to lay in bed, but this actually makes us worse. Bed rest keeps us from moving enough to allow an increase in nutrients into the painful area. The increased nutrients moving into the cells is what allows our joints to heal. The unloading aspect of the water often allows people who can't exercise on land, because of pain, to get the motion that the joints need.

In addition to the joint health benefits, aquatics also build muscle. Muscles support our joints and improve our functional abilities, such as getting up from a chair or stepping up a curb. Any motion performed on land has air resistance, but the same motion underwater is more challenging due to the density of water providing increased resistance. The resistance can be easily increased in the water as progress is made by simply increasing the surface area or adding buoyant resistance (like dumbbells made for water).

All of the movements in the water encourage improved cardiovascular and pulmonary health so you won't be as short of breath with normal activities. These benefits make aquatics great for everyone.

However, aquatic exercise is even more beneficial for anyone with any kind of edema such as Lipedema or Lymphedema because it can help reduce the edema. Every inch of water provides increased pressure or gradiated pressure, so when standing or floating in water the greatest pressure is at the feet and the least pressure is at the surface of the water. This pressure can help decrease edema.

There are many ways to help control edema such as by wearing compression garments and using pumps. But my favorite part about aquatic exercise is that at the same time you receive the benefit of gradiated pressure by being in the water you can also enjoy greater freedom of movement as gravity is nearly eliminated. So, while getting the benefit of compression you can also improve your strength, cardiovascular, pulmonary, and joint health instead of being stuck laying down in a compression pump.

About LaNese Cummings

LaNese Cummings has been a physical therapist since 1997. She loves physical therapy because it provides the opportunity to help people achieve their maximum functional potential. She enjoys working with people of all ages and encouraging them through the rehabilitation process.

Mrs. Cummings provides patients with the tools they need to make and maintain progress by educating them on stretches, therapeutic exercise, and activity modification to promote health and wellbeing. She has spent many years improving manual therapy skills including muscle-energy techniques, functional techniques, mobilizations, and soft tissue massage. Additionally, she is experienced in numerous modalities such as aquatics, taping, wound care management, preventative care, and post-surgical rehabilitation.

She received her bachelor's degree in physical therapy from the University of Oklahoma Health Sciences Center in 1997.

AQUA THERAPY FOR LIPEDEMA AND LYMPHEDEMA

"Water is the mother of the vine, the nurse and fountain of fecundity, the adorner and refresher of the world."

~ Charles Mackay ~

Why Aqua Therapy?

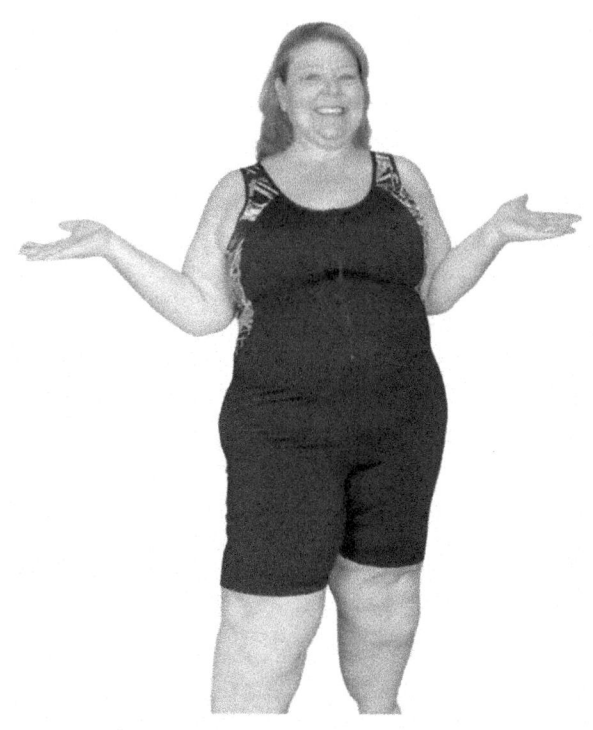

Why Aqua therapy?

Aqua therapy can be several different things: walking or running underwater, exercising in water, aqua cycling, using an underwater treadmill, standing in water and moving the water in patterns towards the body, cold water immersion and even alternating between hot and cold water in the shower. And it can be called many things with varying ways to say "water" and "therapy."

For the purposes of this book, we'll focus on taking advantage of the natural compression, resistance, and support provided by water by walking, jogging or running in water, doing exercises alone or with a group, massage to move lymphatic fluid, deep breathing and gentle stretching in water. I lump this altogether by using the words, "swim" or "aqua therapy" throughout the book.

What I won't cover are cold and hot water treatments that you sometimes see professional athletes using on TV or YouTube, supervised by a professional, because I haven't experienced the benefits of this yet personally or focused my research literature review on relevant information in this area. (Maybe someday!) But for now, swimming and aqua therapy provide more than enough to make a huge difference in our lives as people affected with lipedema or lymphedema!

Swimming is such a refreshing, enjoyable, and empowering way to move our bodies and get exercise. And water is the worst enemy of swelling! Being in the water is one of the best things you can do for a lipedema and lymphedema-affected body simply because it is very easy to be compliant with water exercise, where a lot of other types of self-care are often not adhered to. There are research studies that show patients will stick with aqua therapies more than other conservative treatments like bandaging, wearing compression garments or using pumps to help keep lymphatic fluid moving and swelling down. I believe people stick with swimming because it's easy to do, fun, and freeing.

Water's Natural Compression

At the root of our swelling, we experience with lymphedema and lipedema is that the interstitial / lymphatic fluids are not pumping back to where they should be – which is in the lymphatics, moving their way back to the heart to be reused as body fluids. For whatever reason, like leaky lymphatics, cells that won't release the fluid, a blockage, etc., the lymph fluid is hanging out where it doesn't belong, in our legs, feet, arms, hands or abdomen. So, a key component of managing lymphedema and lipedema is to get the fluid back where it should be. (I'm really oversimplifying the science here.)

To keep swelling at bay, lymph fluid drainage and body movement to help pump the fluid around, are key to managing lipedema and lymphedema. Our ultimate goal is to keep swelling down, so that we can feel less pain, remain mobile, maintain a good range of motion, and definitely not worsen the situation by having fibrosis develop where the lymph has been stuck for a while.

When you move in the water the turbulence of the water combines with movement, and the lymph nodes get activated to help the fluid move up and out of your swollen limbs. The hydrostatic pressure of water helps push the lymph fluid along so it's not staying in the areas of swelling as it gently massages our skin with the movement of water.

There are numerous studies showing that, aqua therapy can significantly reduce limb volume in lymphedema in very few sessions, sometimes in the first session.

Swimming and Aqua therapy Are Good for our Mental Health!

Being in the water feels good to our bodies and refreshes our spirit. Water is a mood booster! Water is proven to relax and relieve anxiety. For those of us who may be feeling pain when we try to exercise on dry land, the joy of being able to freely move with the buoyancy of water and the load of gravity reduced, it can be so nice to be able to move freely without (or with less) pain as we are gently supported by the water, so our backs and knees aren't doing all the work. You weigh a sixth of your dry land body weight in the water, so moving is much easier than on dry land. Then add endorphins generated when we exercise anywhere on top! All of these things improve our mental health.

Finally, taking an active part in owning our physical health by swimming or other activity brings back a sense of control, also improving our mental health and wellbeing.

Physical Benefits of Aqua therapy

Later, we'll have an in-depth look at the natural compression that water provides. There are a lot of facts you need to see, based on research that can help us understand. In general, though the pressure of water (hydrostatic pressure) helps reduce vascular resistance and increases venous return. And blood absorbs oxygen under these pressure conditions well, so blood flow is better overall when our bodies are just in the water. And then we add movement to improve strength and cardiovascular status, and BAM! We have a magical combination.

Exercising in the water can help us to improve balance and flexibility. And when we exercise in the water, we can get stronger and build cardio endurance. For example, I can jog for a solid fifteen minutes in the water and not realize how much time has gone by, especially when I have some good music going by the pool and am just having fun. And sometimes I cannot even believe that it's helping my body way more than if I'd tried something like this on dry land (I wouldn't!). It would tear up my knees and my back would be hurting like crazy if I tried a jog on the street. But in water, I can just...jog, or run, or dance and it just glorious and easy, and I'm also getting resistance from the water, which makes me stronger too. Yes, even if it feels 'easy' water therapy is real exercise.

You can increase your core muscles doing water exercise, taking advantage of the drag and resistance as you move. We can take our time to work on the form while we learn how to move in the water, and can focus on slow controlled movements, relaxation and deep breathing. And while we're learning, we're enjoying the drag and resistance of water, and getting those natural compression benefits.

Water exercise is low impact, so it's great for folks with sore joints, arthritis, or even joint replacements. Swimming is freeing and wonderful. Sometimes when I'm in the water I like to imagine I'm a dancer, and I feel like a kid again as I do fake choreography moves and secret belly dances. Hey! No one can see your moves anyway, so go for it!

And for those of us who've had experiences like I did, where I tried lifting weights, to have someone literally run across the gym, yelling, "stop! You're going to hurt yourself!" It's nice to not worry about hurting yourself on equipment or be embarrassed by lack of knowledge. No one cares if you mess up or modify exercises or sit them out. There's no competition in aqua therapy, unless it's you against your own progress.

In the numerous research studies I've reviewed for this book, I found that aqua therapy was proven to be a safe, effective method for improving measurement of edema, functional level, quality of life, as well social and future concerns for the study participants. The studies also showed that range of motion for affected limbs were improved at a clinically relevant amount with a water exercise program done just **two** times a week. Aqua therapy has physical and mental benefits, can be fun and freeing, and it will help our lipedema and lymphedema swelling.

If we can get ourselves in the water, we can reclaim ownership of our bodies, and add another tool in our arsenal of managing lipedema and lymphedema while adding a little fun and freedom too!

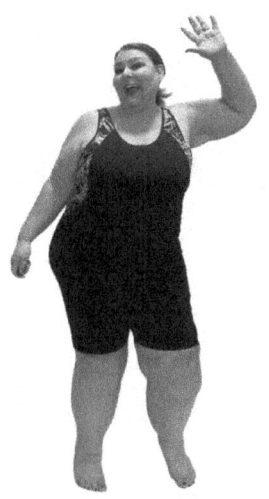

"All water is holy water."

~ Rajiv Joseph ~

My Story

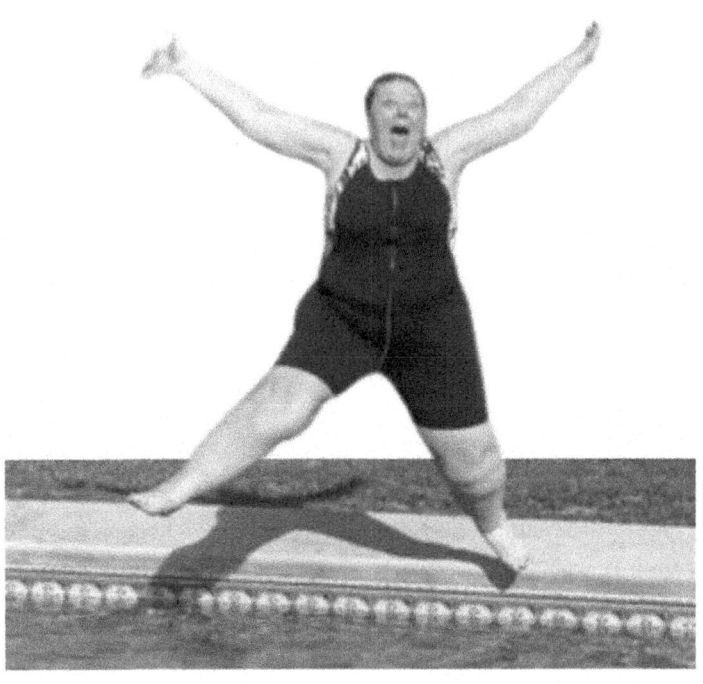

Chapter 1: My Story

Note: I'm re-sharing some information about my story that I originally wrote for <u>Jeans on a Beach Day</u> (my first book), for the benefit of folks who may not have read it. I've added a bit of an update to that original story to talk about my experiences with aqua therapy since I put in a pool and spent a great deal of time in the water and in performing an intensive literature of papers on the topic.

I love the water, always have. Even when there were times when my legs didn't look so great out by the ocean or walking around a beach town while wearing shorts, I loved every minute I could be near water. In my first book, <u>Jeans on A Beach Day</u>, I tell the story of how it took me years of thinking I might have cancer before I discovered I had lipo-lymphedema and that through a series of events, was able to receive surgical intervention to remove nodules and fibrous, diseased tissue. I begin implementing therapies like wearing compression to help me try to avoid swelling to keep my condition from progressing from a stage three lipo-lymphedema to a stage four or beyond.

I've been overweight since about second grade and suffered all the things that kids do to each other because of it. I was on the grapefruit diet by age eight. I was a pretty active and outdoorsy kid, but always the one wearing husky jeans. Years of different diets and shenanigans with my body left me, done with it all until I had kids. Or at least until I wanted to have kids.

My fertility struggle has to fit into this whole mix somewhere. For several years during the time, I was trying to get pregnant, I went to several doctors for help. This time was incredibly difficult psychologically. I experienced numerous doctors who fat shamed me, told me I wasn't healthy enough to have a child, told me to lose weight, and even who told me that their medical equipment and speculums weren't long enough for me to be treated. So not only was I already self-conscious about my body, but I began to think of myself as not even a normal or real woman because I couldn't bear children. I eventually found a who not only immediately recognized that I had polycystic ovary syndrome (PCOS) but was able to find the right treatment that helped me to get pregnant two months after I started his treatment plan.

I left the hospital after delivering my first child with legs that would never be the same as they were before pregnancy. After several months on fertility hormones and then being prescribed progesterone for a total of 12 months during pregnancies, my legs had developed into "tree trunks." Also, I'd had a blood clot develop in my groin in late pregnancy and had to have surgery to repair it two weeks before my delivery date. Unfortunately, I experienced significant physical trauma during the vaginal birth when the clot's repair site that hadn't healed fully, burst, and had to be repaired right there in the childbirth suite. This clot, and scars damaged my lymphatics, and ultimately caused me to develop lymphedema in my left leg on top of the lipedema that had formed.

With the birth of my second child (and another round of hormones to get there) the lipedema in my legs worsened, and they grew even more. I continued to work full time in a professional management position, incurring significant chronic stress while raising the kids with my husband. A few years later I noticed nodules that felt like painful golf balls under my skin especially behind my knees and on my calves, as the stress in my job increased dramatically. I believed I was developing cancerous tumors in my legs.

I had natively started wearing maxi dresses to cover my legs and had one day - years ago - decided shorts as a regular outfit piece weren't for me and had also switched to wearing long men's board shorts over my bathing suit to hide the growing bulges. I felt jealous when I saw women my age, some of whom were bigger than me, who still had nice legs to show off when all I wanted was to cover mine to the floor. I somehow felt, 'less than,' because I couldn't get my legs under control, despite having bariatric surgery twice and losing more than 150 pounds, training and completing a (walking) half marathon, and enjoying being an active mother. I simply did not understand what was going on with my body.

My legs had been growing for a while and the backs of my calves especially got very hard and fibrotic. The fibrosis in my left (lymphedema) leg was particularly advanced, with the entire inside of my calf staying firm. When I moved to wiggle it, my calf moved in one big, solid piece, instead of jiggling like normal fat. My legs even developed lumps so large that I'd named them.

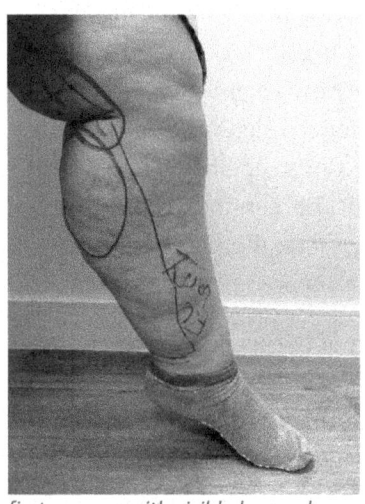

My leg right before my first surgery with visible lumps, bumps and hard tissue there.

My primary doctor at home was very kind and worked with me extensively to try and figure out what was going on as each new symptom appeared. She sent me for x-rays, blood work, and several MRIs, but the results were inconclusive. The two of us had all but given up and explored alternatives including switching to a vegetarian diet for several years and even considered a third bariatric surgery which, I thankfully, decided not to do. Although they were well meaning, none of these treatments helped my condition. My legs even continued to grow while I was a dedicated vegetarian! I saw my trusted physical therapist to see if she had any tricks to reducing, 'Larry' (the name I had given to the large lump on my left calf), but neither of us knew what it was at the time.

I suffered for years with legs that ached constantly and kept me awake at night. When my cats walked on me, it hurt deeply. I tried all kinds of things to help: creams, ace bandages, icing, fascia blasting, rolling them with a rolling pin, special exercises and targeted weightlifting. Sadly, the only results were wasted time and money, and a lot of strange bruises that looked like I had been beaten severely in the legs.

One day, I developed a sudden bout of tendonitis in my foot, rendering me nearly immobile. I saw a foot specialist, who sent me to a brace company to have a special brace fitted before a trip to New York with my Girl Scouts that would require miles of walking each day. I was only in my mid-forties and not ready to quit doing fun things like this. I was determined to use the brace and take the trip.

At the brace supplier, the technician casually asked me, "Who is treating your lymphedema?" Lymphedema? I had never heard of this word. It had a name. And there were other people around who were hiding their legs and suffering like me? Total lightbulb moment!

I went back to my doctor and reported what the brace technician had said. She immediately sent me to a certified lymphedema specialist for decongestive therapy. The therapist assigned me swimming therapy, arranged for me to get a pneumatic compression pump, and taught me about bandaging my legs to reduce them, and helped me with compression.

I was angry at having gone years of not knowing that my condition was legitimate or special or real, but I was also relieved, finally, to have a sense of understanding about what was happening to my body. I had hope that I could get the swelling down enough to wear a pair of shorts again maybe someday with some dignity.

I saw the therapist faithfully several times a week, was measured for compression, bought boxes and loads of bandages / wrapping supplies, started using my pneumatic pump daily, and began to see some differences in the size of my legs.

The goal of all these treatments was just to reduce the swelling and inflammation, and then the compression was to keep it from coming back. I was to wear the bandage wraps for 24-36 hours at a time and take them off only to shower or to be rewrapped. I struggled with wearing wraps on my legs because they slid down quite easily, it's hard to walk with them on, and they're bulky, and so on. I opted to purchase Velcro ready wraps instead. The first ones I bought were customizable, and my therapist cut them down to fit me perfectly. After I wore this type for a while, I discovered other wraps available on Amazon that were constructed multiple layers of Velcro and could be adjusted each time they were put on. So as swelling changed my leg size, I could still use the same wraps. Also, I was able to wear these wraps on top of leggings or compression, and I could move! Best of all, they were effective in reducing my swelling!

My new lymphedema diagnosis led me to join multiple Facebook support groups for lymphedema patients. Just when things were starting to feel better and I thought I was at the end of the line for treatment, both of my legs flared up with almost double the normal swelling and pain levels and went out of control, correlating with a ridiculously stressful day at work. In a single day, several new bumpy and painful golf ball sized nodules appeared out of nowhere.

I went to every resource I knew including my newly found online support groups, asking for help once again. When I shared photos of my legs online, I learned from some of my new friends that I may have actually had late-stage lipedema (lipo-lymphedema). Never having heard the word lipedema, I went down another rabbit hole of research and for the first time, I saw so many people with legs like mine on the internet! I immediately felt a kindred spirit with these brave souls who had shared their pictures and helped me figure it all out. It was the <u>pictures</u> that explained so much. Epiphany! Finally, I had a term to Google, and a way to connect with specialists knowledgeable with the conditions I was experiencing.

Through the internet, I connected with a doctor specializing in lipedema who looked at my pictures remotely and had me fill out a very extensive questionnaire, providing a very thorough history on my legs. His office also gathered information on my mother's legs. Hers looked like mine too but without the lymphedema component that I'd gotten from the traumatic childbirth experience. After receiving my documentation and family history, I met with the doctor and his staff over the phone to begin my journey towards treatment. Four years after I started my search in earnest, I finally received a written diagnosis by Dr. Jaime Schwartz in California, halfway across the country. Lipedema.

Once I got the diagnosis, I moved extremely fast to get surgical treatment – I'm not getting any younger and I have so much to do! I switched insurance companies to one that is known to cover lipedema. I gathered all my documentation including test results and scans over the years, my receipts from treatments and purchases to date, and got my package ready. I was approved for surgery in January 2021, and by mid-February 2021, I was laying on the operating table in Beverly Hills and had the first 16 liters of lipedema tissue removed. I documented my surgical recoveries every step of the way on my YouTube channel (youtube.com/c/LegsLikeMine) so maybe I could help someone plan for recovery as they went through similar surgery.

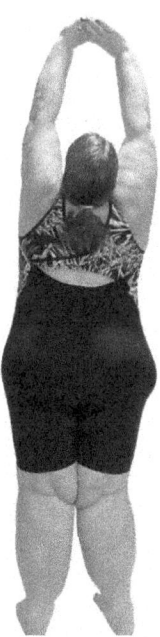

As of the writing of this book, I've had three surgeries with Dr. Schwartz to help get my legs under control. Since these initial treatments, I continue to wear compression and wraps regularly, swim, and receive regular lymphatic therapy. Yes, my legs are still lumpy and bumpy, and they swell (I still have lipo-lymphedema), but they don't hurt as much as they used to. I wear swimming suits, shorts, and shorter dresses than I have in twenty years. Most importantly, I'm able to walk without pain again after years of suffering. I deal with significant lymphedema in my left leg, especially when I fly or take long road trips. I've added a new Fast N' Go bandage set to my arsenal of tools and use them on my worst nights to wrap when everything else I have to throw at lipo-lymphedema isn't enough.

Since I've started sharing my story, I've helped thousands of people with questions and connections related to lipedema and lymphedema. I'm committed to feverishly overshare and give support online with many people in various stages of the treatment and diagnosis journey. I feel very deeply that I, and you, need to do what we can to share our stories so others can receive diagnoses in time to save their mobility and dignity.

Along my journey I've learned that millions of women have lipedema and millions more men and women have lymphedema, and that I'm not a freak or rarity, but part of a big percentage of the population. There is some debate about the studies, but several sources, including the National Institutes of Health website cite that 11% of women have lipedema. ELEVEN PERCENT.

Through becoming part of the lipedema and lymphedema, and hypermobility communities, I've accepted the conditions I have to be part of me, and now believe that I do indeed fit in. And yes, I'm still pretty. It took a lot of time, but I'm at peace with where I am. I'm honestly just glad to know that I have a real disease and that I'm not a failure for not being able to get my legs to slim down through diets and exercise. I even feel like it's appropriate and right to continue doing things I love like snorkeling, playing on the beach, hiking and camping, and to show my legs more. It helps other people feel comfortable too when they see other imperfect people enjoying life. I carry little cards about lipedema that I can discretely share with women who look like me. I know I would be forever grateful back in the day when I had no clue what was going on, to even know the word lipedema.

I hear over and over that doctors receive only one hour of training on the lymphatic system during medical school. My experience is that lipedema and lymphedema, while not rare, are very rarely diagnosed correctly. Diagnosing as early as possible is imperative to slow progression with conservative treatments. This is another reason why we need to be aggressively sharing the story. Many of us, including myself, had doctors who hadn't been trained to recognize and diagnose lipedema. Others, sadly, have doctors who diagnose it as obesity, and worse, some who fat shame.

If we can get more doctors aware of the disease, we can get to needed treatment. Because of this I've been very willing and open to share my story with my medical team. Before my experience, my friend and physical therapist and my occupational therapist had had experience with lymphedema but not lipedema. Working with them increased their medical knowledge and awareness as they supported me. And now that has helped them treat and recognize lipedema in other patients they see and to share my little compression things I've been successful at with others as well.

As I mentioned, I decided to get courageous and share my story -- well, actually OVER share my story. I started adding pictures to Instagram and Facebook, began blogging on LegsLikeMine.com, and started educating any medical professional who touches me about my condition, including my dentist! I brought pamphlets from the Lipedema Foundation to my doctor, let other doctors and therapists touch and feel my legs to familiarize themselves with the feel of the nodules in them, and invited my occupational therapist to have her peers come and see me before and after surgery. I started referring other lipedema patients to my medical team, both at home and in California. Additionally, I answered (and continue to) thousands of emails and messages from desperate women, all searching for the name of their disease and a way to receive treatment, wanting to know what I've experienced, and asking for advice, help, or just a listening ear.

After answering many questions individually, but repeatedly to different people, (and with the guidance of my husband who is a prolific blogger), I learned that capturing my knowledge and experiences in blog format was a more efficient way to share the same information with multiple people asking the same questions. So now when a frequently asked question comes my way, I am able to simply share a link to a blog post answering a question on that topic.

Since writing of <u>Jeans on a Beach Day</u>, we put in a pool for exercise, and I've become a self-made expert in the aqua therapy moves that feel good to me. And now that I've spent literally hundreds of hours researching studies on aqua therapy for various conditions, I feel it is my duty to roll what I've learned together into a book to share with you. This stuff is just too good!

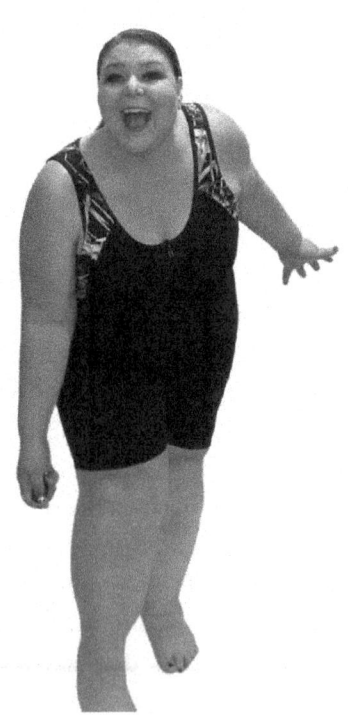

I get in my pool as often as I can in the unpredictable Oklahoma weather. The pool is heated, so I swim year-round. I've also been fortunate to retire from my stressful job that had me on planes several times a month. This now allows me the time I need to rest, swim, and attend physical and occupational therapy as frequently as I need to. I still attend YMCA classes for water exercise and good energy vibes. I like being in the company of the class, the energy and guidance of the instructors, and the fun music for Water Zumba. And I continue to pursue water sports like snorkeling, which is my personal favorite (but just now in cleaner water than the brown waters of Oklahoma). Sorry, if I have to go to Hawaii, I guess I'll go!

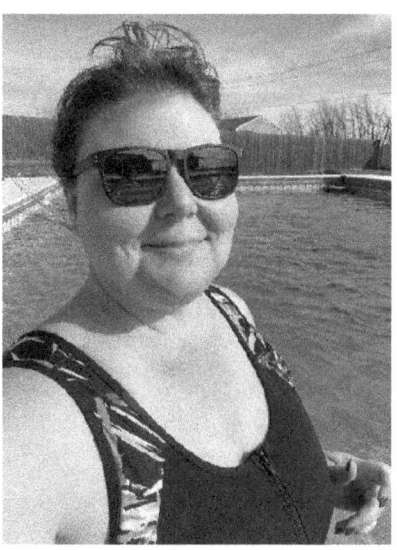

I hope my experiences and time dedicated to researching will help just one person improve their physical and mental health, help one more person have less pain, or one more person be less afraid of wearing a suit in public to get to the water that is so beneficial for us. Enjoy the book and feel free to reach out to me at LegsLikeMine@gmail.com. Let me know what's working and not working for you so we can all keep learning together!

"Water links us to our neighbor in a way more profound and complex than any other."

~ John Thorson ~

What are Lipedema and Lymphedema?

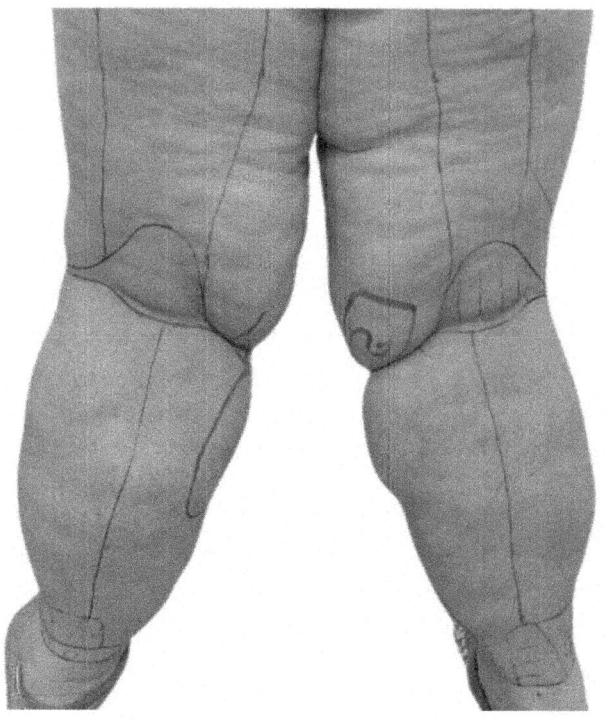

Chapter 2: What are Lipedema, Lymphedema and Fibrosis?

You may be wondering why this book is about two unique conditions, lipedema, and lymphedema. The root causes of lipedema aren't fully known, but advanced stages of lipedema develop into what's called lipo-lymphedema, where both conditions are present. They are linked together.

Both conditions have the need to move interstitial and lymphatic fluids through the body more efficiently to reduce swelling. And research shows both can benefit from aqua therapy. What I've observed through reading is that many research papers tended to focus on one condition. When we combine the research together, we can get a good picture of the potential benefits of aqua therapy for both lipedema and lymphedema.

Lipedema

Lipedema is a genetic disease that causes the body to distribute fat in an irregular way below the skin. It affects mostly women. Many doctors and researchers believe that with lipedema, fat distributes symmetrically between legs and buttocks, but many women also have it in different representations including their arms and bellies, and even asymmetrically.

Symptoms of lipedema include having large legs that sometimes look like tree trunks and don't turn in towards the ankle like more typical legs. They can be lumpy or bumpy or hard and fibrotic depending on the stage of lipedema. Some women just have big bums or very large arms. Some have big thighs with small calves, while others have big calves and small thighs. There are many types and stages.

Several good websites like **lipedema.com**, have fantastic amounts of research complete with pictures, and detailed medical information on the disease. Before you look at my pictures and decide you don't have lipedema because you're not shaped exactly like me, please visit these professional sites to see the types and stages of lipedema. The manifestation of the disease is quite diverse.

QR Link to the Lipedema.com area that discusses lipedema and lymphedema.

As lipedema progresses, the appearance of cuffing can occur by the ankles and at the wrists, like folds of fat are hanging over the ankle and wrists. In later stages of lipedema, lymphedema can also develop and then leakage of lymphatic fluid happens, hard skin growths, and immobility occur due to the enormous weight of the overgrown lipidemic areas and damage to joints.

The following picture shows what my legs looked like on a trip to Savannah, GA prior to being diagnosed with even lymphedema, or having lipedema removal surgery. The left leg is definitely displaying more lymphedema, and the right leg has a pitting edema near the top of the calf. This was the trip where everyone began wondering, "What the heck is wrong with Susan's legs?" This was also the first time in my life I opted to not put on a swimming suit and get in the water at the amazing Tybee

Island beach, later that same day. It's a sad memory for me, even though I am walking down the streets of Savannah wearing a pirate hat!

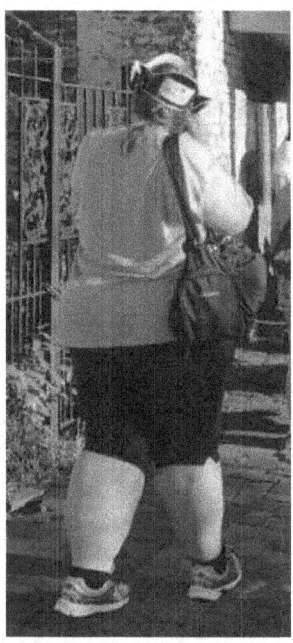

The first day I opted to not put on a swimsuit in front of others. A sad day for me. And this is a fantastic picture of Lipo-Lymphedema.

Other symptoms of lipedema include pain in the fat. For me personally, it hurt when I was in a seat that was even slightly too small, and sometimes even with just a seatbelt being on me. My legs and knees throbbed in bed every night. Another symptom is easy bruising. Many of us suffering with lipedema regularly develop 'mystery bruises' all over the affected areas. Having been a very frequent traveler for more than twenty years, I could always count on receiving mystery bruises on travel days, moving days, and sometimes even laundry days, and the bruises would last for weeks.

For many, we have lipedema nodules in the affected area. Mine varied in size; some were as small as grains of rice, with others larger than a golf ball. I had nodules in my calves, behind my knees, inside my thighs, and in my upper arms. My doctor eventually removed many of them with a special liposuction technique, but I still have several yet to be removed, and several still growing in size. Those nodules, again for me, were incredibly painful, and doctors could easily feel them by simple palpation. One of my nodules (the one named "Larry") I felt was visible from across the street. When I see this picture now, I want to just grab the massive fat pads inside my knees and pull them off. I wish it had been that easy!

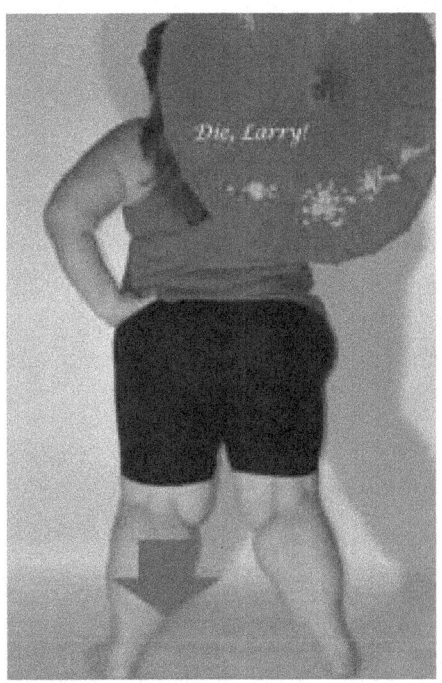

"Larry," the ever-present and growing nodule inside my left calf. It swelled to 'amazing' proportions during times of stress, and it hurt deeply at night.

All of these areas are resistant to traditional diet and exercise. For many, again like me, bariatric surgery would take away the normal adipose/fat tissue, but the lipedema legs remain along with a disappointed patient who's more than likely gone through quite a bit to qualify for bariatric surgery, not knowing that a portion of her 'fat' is lipedema that will remain despite reduction in calories and smaller stomach size.

The next picture is a golf ball sized nodule (one of many) on the inside of my right knee prior to any surgeries for removal. The nodules on the inside of my knees called 'fat pads' are especially concerning. These pads push my knees outward. After time, it stretched the connective tissues in my knees permanently. My mobility was affected before surgery because they rubbed together and hurt deeply – down to the bone. And after surgery, I now have the hypermobile knees due to the loose and stretched connective tissues. So, after surgery my knees dislocate sideways quite frequently, especially when they aren't pushing directly down by my standing. So, lipedema is a double whammy. Again, getting treatment early can help save the fat pads from growing, which helps the knee tissues from stretching, so you don't dislocate all the time.

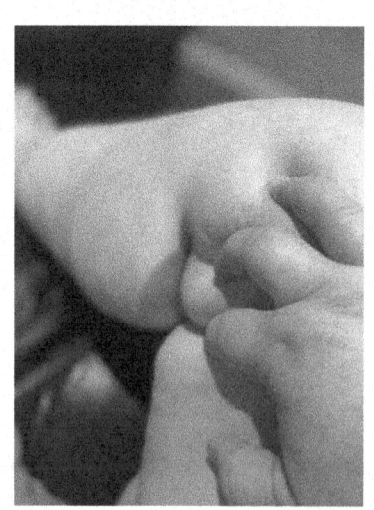

Golf ball sized nodule on my right medial knee.

The next picture shows what my legs looked like after I had had my first bariatric surgery and lost 167 pounds in 2007. You can see lipedema in both legs and lymphedema in the left, with it being quite a bit larger than the other. By then I'd already had both of my children using fertility treatments and was age 34. I was eating very small amounts of only protein and walking up to fourteen miles a day to stay at this weight. My hair was falling out and I was perpetually fatigued. Also, I was a hungry mama and I really missed most of the food I used to enjoy, including even vegetables. You can still see quite a bit of fibrosis in my legs, and folds and fat pads in the knee area. I promise you; this is as skinny as my body can be. And it only lasted for a very short time as I could not continue starving and having to work out that much.

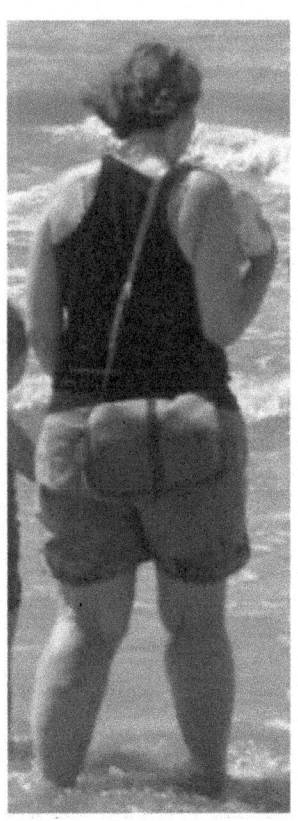

Lipedema and Lymphedema still present after my 167 lb. weight loss.

One thing to reiterate is that lipedema takes many forms. While it heavily affected my legs, arms, and belly, for some women it manifests in the hips and buttocks only, or in certain areas of the legs and arms, or any combination of these. There is also the lymphedema component in later stages of lipedema, which complicates getting a good diagnosis.

There are several websites, such as lipedema.org (the Lipedema Foundation), that have pictures of different manifestations of lipedema. They also have a brochure that you can download or order for sharing with medical professionals and other women that describes lipedema. I've referred many people to this website and am so grateful for The Lipedema Foundation's work.

If you're like me and many women who suspect they have lipedema, you'll want to dig into the best research around ad you'll find there is a lot of self-care involved in its management. If there is one document that I'd suggest you read, it would be the Standard of Care for Lipedema in the United States, designed to, "advance our understanding towards early diagnosis, treatments, and ultimately a cure for affected individuals." This is the ground-breaking consensus document, led by Dr. Karen Herbst, who is a premier researcher and speaker on lipedema. This document is the one that we should refer to when working with insurance companies and doctors when they need convincing that lipedema is real and needs to be treated properly and aggressively. I have a citation to it in the bibliography section of this book and a QR code below – it's that important.

QR Link to the Standard of Care for Lipedema in the United States.

What Causes Lipedema?

Recent research is showing that lipedema rears its ugly head at time of hormonal changes in women and that it is indeed genetic.

Puberty, hormone ingestion, pregnancy, and menopause may trigger its onset, but allow me to reiterate that any woman suffering with lipedema did not do anything to cause it. For many sufferers including myself, stress (which releases cortisol into the system) can cause affected areas to flare up as well.

Within the last six years, researchers have begun publishing more information on lipedema than ever before. These papers and studies have shown a possible genetic biomarker for lipedema. And once they've found the genetic cause, the next step is research on a medicine that can prevent or reverse its effects. If you or your daughters are suffering from lipedema, hang in there! In our lifetimes, there could be a medicinal cure and even prevention for the disease. Until that happens, we'll have to go with the treatments available and do as much as we can on our own to avoid disease progression. Aqua therapy can be an important and effective part of this self-management.

If there's one thing you need to take away from this chapter, it's this: *lipedema is genetic*. Read that again, to yourself. You did not cause your lipedema. You don't deserve it and you couldn't have prevented it. It is not your fault. But it is your job to manage it to avoid progression so you can live the best life possible.

Lymphedema

While lymphedema can exist as a single condition, it is also related to lipedema in that lipedema progresses to lipo-lymphedema in its later stages where lymphedema is present in addition to lipedema. Both conditions need to be managed similarly to avoid progression, and can benefit from treatments like wearing compression, and both can benefit from participating in aqua therapy.

Lymphedema is a condition that causes swelling in parts of the body, often the arms or legs, but it can be anywhere, including the genitals, breasts, face, etc. It's caused by a buildup of lymph fluid in the fatty tissues under the skin. Like lipedema, early identification and treatment might prevent progression of the disease and make your quality of life better.

A good resource for finding more information about lymphedema is the May Clinic Website. I've added a QR code here for you to connect with them easily. (I use the Mayo clinic for a TON of research).

QR Link to the Mayo Clinic's topic on Lymphedema Diagnosis and Treatment

What Causes Lymphedema?

Lymphedema is caused when the lymph system is damaged, before, during, or after birth. Some people are born with it (primary lymphedema), and some get it from damage that occurs after a person is born (secondary lymphedema). Regardless of whether it is primary or secondary, damage keeps lymph fluid from flowing properly and pumping back into the blood supply. Things like cancer surgery where lymph nodes are affected or removed, radiation, infections, injury or trauma, or even leukemia can be some of the causes of lymphedema.

People who have lymphedema might have swelling, tightness, aching, loss of flexibility in joints that are nearby. Clothing and jewelry might get tight in the affected area. If it's not treated, lymphedema can become very serious and develop into weeping, extreme pain, development of large lobules, cellulitis, infections, or some cancers, and worse.

The goal of lipedema treatment is to help us to live a normal life. Just like with lipedema, that means managing pain, staying mobile with flexibility and full range of motion, reducing inflammation, keeping the lymphatic flow going, making sure you are mentally, emotionally and spiritually cared for, and finally preventing development of lobules, fibrosis, and infections..

Fibrosis

Fibrosis occurs in the body if inflammation is in an area of the body for an extended period and causes scar tissue to form by leaving too much collagen in the swollen area. The collagen forms into tough fibrous tissues. Depending on where the fibrous tissue is made, it can limit mobility, be painful and disfiguring. So, fibrosis is a direct result of swelling and inflammation that can be caused by lipedema and lymphedema.

The fibrous areas are what patients like me, who had significant areas of hard scar tissue, have removed surgically. The surgery turns back time but doesn't remove the genes causing lipedema or the trauma to lymphatics that could have caused lymphedema. And sadly, not all people with lipedema or lymphedema are covered by insurance or can afford or have access to surgical intervention. It takes an investment of both time and money. Keep in mind that surgery is not a cure, and you will need to continue wearing compression, moving, and eating well for life in order for it to keep your body in the best condition you can, for as long as you can.

Wearing compression and decongesting the area of swelling are important to keeping swelling at by. So being in compression whether it's in the form of wearing stockings, a sleeve, a custom compression garment, or being in the water, helps prevent progression of lipedema and lymphedema by getting swelling out of the affected areas in the body.

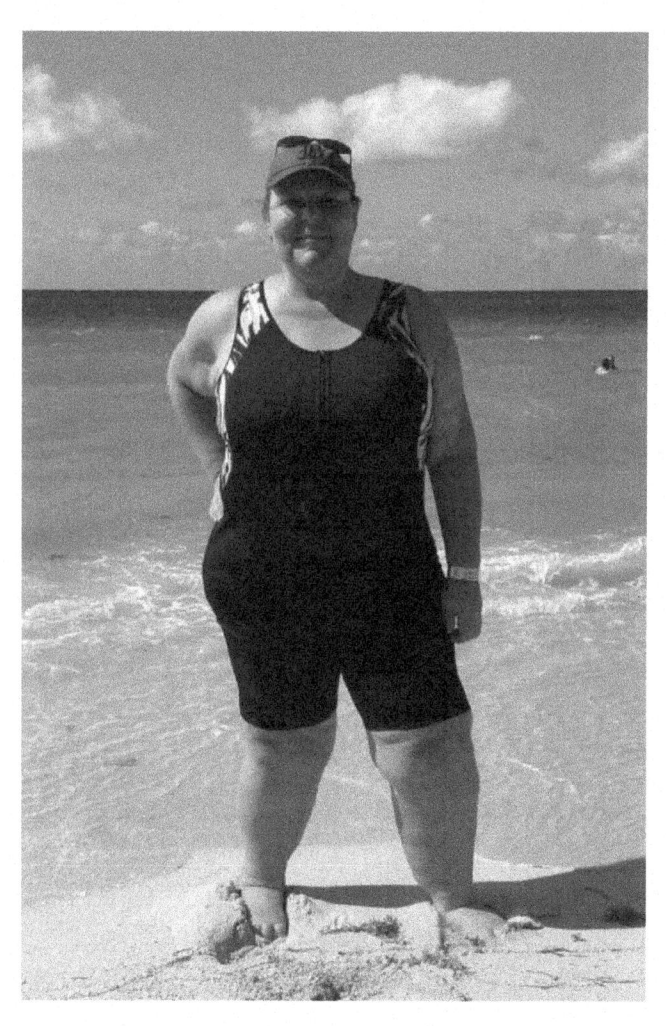

Swimming in Cozumel a few months after my most recent surgery to remove fibrosis and nodules. You can see the lymphedema in my left leg clearly. Water was so good for my soul and my travel-weary legs!

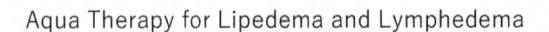

"A river cuts through rock not because of its power but because of its persistence."

~ Jim Watkins ~

Aqua Therapy for Lipedema and Lymphedema

Water is Natural Compression

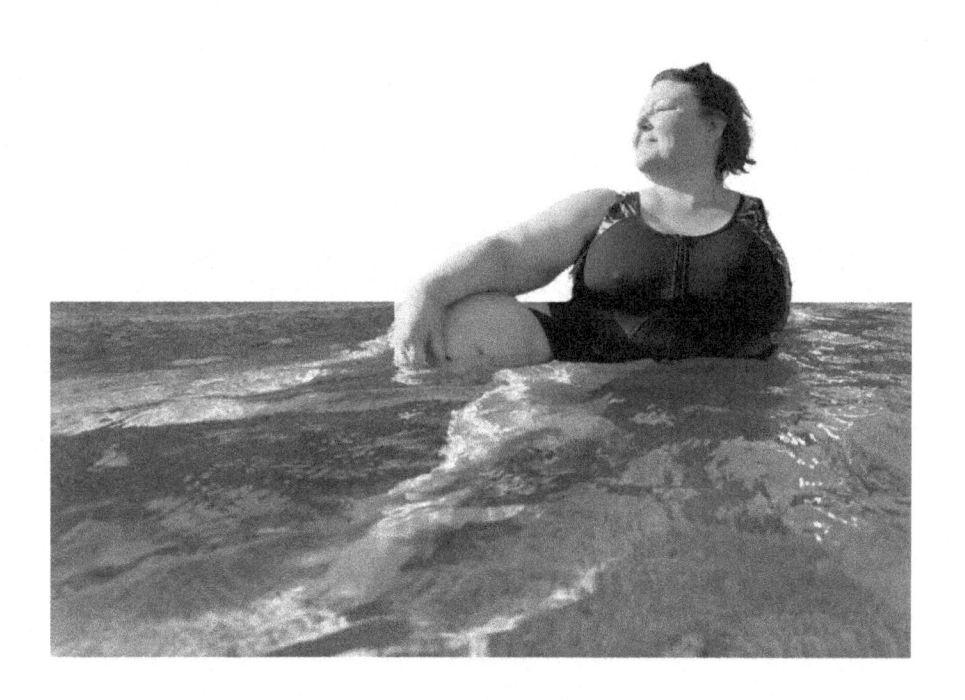

Chapter 3: Water is Natural Compression

Why Compression is Important

So far, we've discussed that compression is an important part of managing lipedema and lymphedema. But why? The reason for this is that the lymphatic system isn't like the circulatory system – there is no heart to pump lymphatic fluid back up and recirculate it.

Compression applies pressure to the body and helps trapped lymph fluid flow through the lymphatic system. Wearing compression gives a little extra oomph, pushing against muscles when they work, which also helps fluid drain. So, moving and compression is better than just wearing compression. Exercise and compression help the lymphatic fluid move about and circulate properly.

A beautiful prescription for lymphatic health would be to tell the patient to move under compression, or to move in water, which provides natural compression and pressure against the muscles to move lymphatic fluid and eliminate swelling.

How Water Compression Measures Up

Compression is measured in millimeters of mercury, denoted as mmHg. Water is heavy, and it provides natural, graduated (more at the feet that the thighs if you're in the water feet-first, for example) compression, which is just what lipedema and lymphedema patients need. A foot of water depth (or around. three meters) gives 22 mmHg of hydrostatic pressure. This is the same amount as a medical grade compression stocking. And most of us swim or walk in water with our feet further down than just one foot! At 4 feet deep, water provides 89 mmHg of pressure. To really simplify this, the deeper you go, the more immersion effects you get by compressing your tissues, and recirculating blood and lymphatic fluids.

And what's great about being in the water is that its compression is coming at you from all sides that are submersed equally at the same depth. A lot of compression garments can't do that, where they might have an opening, or a weakness so the pressure isn't equal, where being in water applies equal pressure.

How do Compression Garments Measure Up

Compression stockings are generally graded by the amount of compression they provide. Naturally, the US, Europe and France all have different grade definitions of compression with slightly different amounts of hydrostatic pressure for each grade. In the US, companies set the compression grading standards, and the government doesn't have an actual set standard, so grades can vary from company to company. There are two main classifications, however, that are similar, AFNOR (Association Française de Normalisation) and RAL (European Union classifications). We're going to use RAL for the purposes of the book.

Classes of Compression

Class 1: 18-21 mmHg compression is Very Light Compression, the lowest grade, typically available over the counter. These may come in knee-high, thigh-high, pantyhose or maternity pantyhose styles.

Class 2: 23-32 mmHg compression is Moderate Compression and are the first medical grade compression stockings. It is the most widely used, providing ample compression without being too strong. These are generally recommended for the treatment of varicose veins, spider veins, leg swelling, and after surgery.

Class 3: 34-46 mmHg compression is Strong Compression. This level is recommended for more serious symptoms. They are also commonly recommended for those with deep vein thrombosis, blood clots, and lymphedema.

Class 4: 49 mmHg and up is Very Strong Compression, which offers the strongest grade of compression. This level of compression is usually reserved for those with severe venous stasis and lymphedema.

Class 1	Class 2	Class 3	Class 4
18-21 mmHg	23-32	34-46	49 and up
Light Compression	Moderate Compression	Strong Compression	Very Strong Compression

RAL, European Union Classification for Compression.

Water Compression vs. Compression Garment Strength

We know how much compression water creates and how much compression is in garments. We can now match depths of water to classes of compression.

Depth/ Compression	How Much Compression Water Provides Equally from All Sides
1 Foot Deep	22.25 mmHg = Class 2 Compression
2 Feet Deep	44.5 mmHg = Class 3 Compression
3 Feet Deep	66.75 mmHg = Class 4 Compression
4 Feet Deep	89 mmHg High End Class 4 Compression
5 Feet Deep	111 mmHg Better than Compression!

The deeper your body is in the water, the more compression it's getting from **all** sides. Often compression garments don't apply equal pressure to all areas, so water is better than just wearing a garment.

**Water is Natural Compression: Hydrostatic Pressure
In Five Feet of Water**

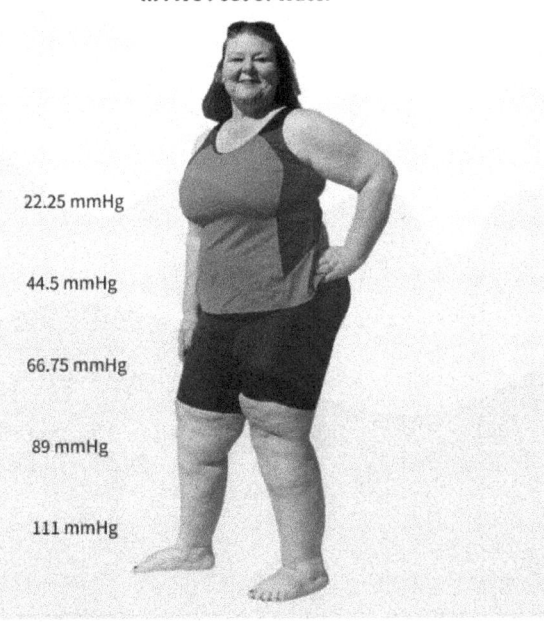

22.25 mmHg

44.5 mmHg

66.75 mmHg

89 mmHg

111 mmHg

*Hydrostatic Pressure in **five** feet of water. My feet would be getting 111 mmHg of pressure when I stand in 5 feet of water, which is neck deep for me. This is stronger than even custom-made medical compression!*

**Water is Natural Compression: Hydrostatic Pressure
In Four Feet of Water**

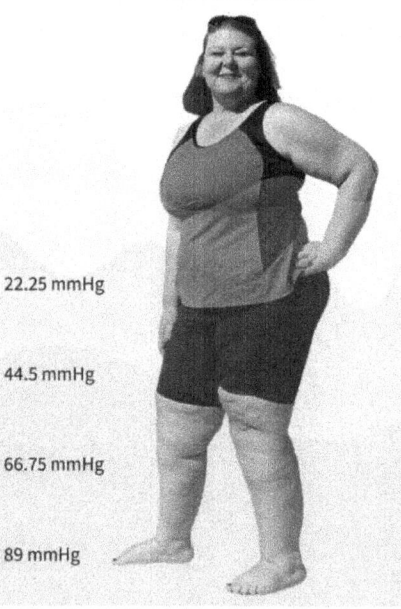

22.25 mmHg

44.5 mmHg

66.75 mmHg

89 mmHg

*Hydrostatic Pressure in **four** feet of water. My feet would be getting 89 mmHg of pressure when I stand in 4 feet of water, which is chest deep for me. This is as strong as Very Strong Class 4, medical-grade compression!*

**Water is Natural Compression: Hydrostatic Pressure
In Three Feet of Water**

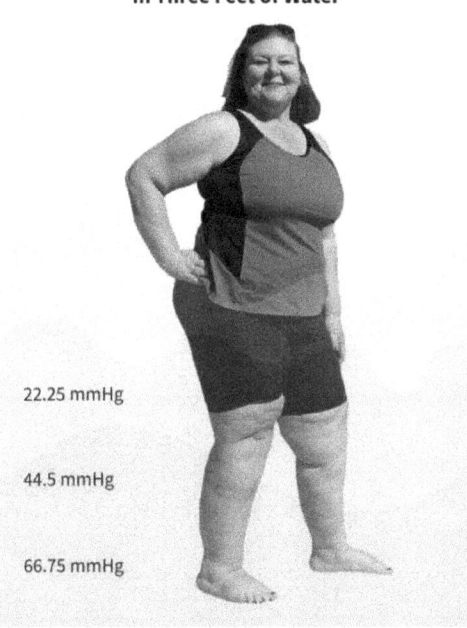

22.25 mmHg

44.5 mmHg

66.75 mmHg

*Hydrostatic Pressure in **three** feet of water. My feet would be getting 66.75 mmHg of pressure when I stand in 3 feet of water, which is low waist deep for me. This is as strong as Class 4, medical-grade compression!*

"Water is the reason of our birth, it is the healer, the destroyer and the final consumer."

~ Neeraj Singhvi ~

Start with Your Mind

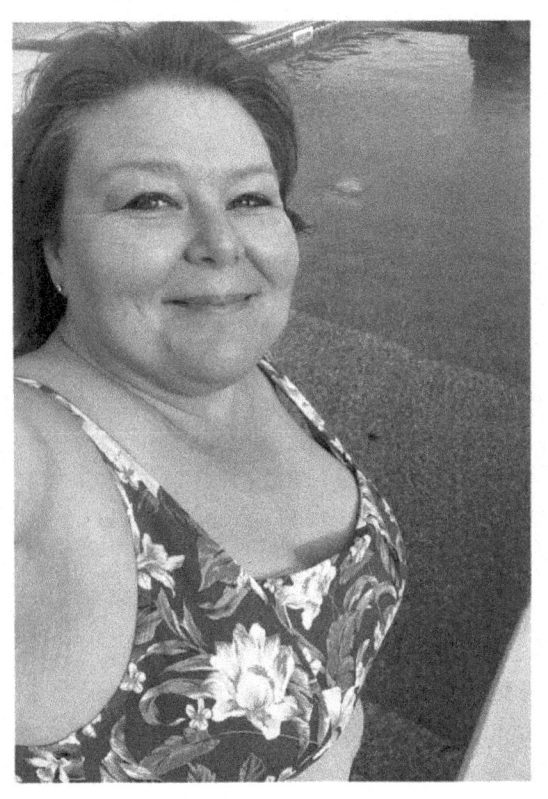

Chapter 4: Aqua therapy Starts with the Mind

It seems like there are so many things that we 'should be doing' like wearing compression, dry brushing, skin care, rebounding, pumping, using vibration plates, walking, performing manual lymphatic drainage, eating well, (and on and on), that it's hard to figure out how to manage our time and our real lives too. What I see in many is that we just give up because it's too overwhelming. And the clinics that provide not only one-time treatments, but continuing care, overseeing medications, swelling management and condition monitoring are practically non-existent. The few that are around are often too far for patients to return to regularly for routine care.

As a result, patients literally have to decide that we are in charge of managing our conditions and set our minds that we're not giving up. One of the first things to tackle as a lipedema or lymphedema patient is the fact that sadly, a lot of the care for managing our disease is self-care and compliance, and it can be overwhelming at times.

The good news is that one thing we know we can do, and enjoy, is to swim and perform aqua therapy. And guess what, we don't have to be at a doctor's office or the occupational therapist's room to make this happen. You can take the tools we will learn in this book anywhere there is a body of water and begin helping yourself!

The most important thing you can do is to make up your mind that you are going to do something, even just one thing, to try and manage your body with lipedema or lymphedema. If you can allow yourself to meet yourself where you are right now, and get in the pool, lake or ocean wearing even street clothes, it's a start. And then literally tell yourself and believe that getting in the water will do you good physically, mentally, and spiritually. You can make a difference in your condition's progression, swelling, and pain by taking this activity on. I truly believe this, and hope you can too.

You may feel discouraged about exercise in general. We patients range from being fairly active, fighting the disease, all the way to being completely bedbound, sometimes due to physical limitations, and sometimes due to our mindsets, after years of dieting, ignorance from medical professionals, and repeated attempts at fixing things to no avail.

For example, I personally know women whose physical conditions are better than my own, but who have decided to lay in the bed. I also personally know women whose conditions are far more progressed than my body is, yet they get up and fight every day with exercise and movement. In fact, some of them lead others in therapeutic activities.

I am respectfully recognizing and validating those who physically are at a place where they cannot exercise any longer. But a lot of how we choose to live with our conditions truly is a mindset. For me, I want to move. I want to live, and I want to try my hardest to have a good life without pain. I do not want to be stuck in a bed. I hope you are able to decide to get out of the bed or off that couch, (you know who you are) and get moving! Because no one else is going to do it for you.

Affirmations

Regardless of where you are in your physical journey, you can help yourself by practicing affirmations. Doing this can activate and literally rewire parts of your brain and then impact how you experience things. Affirmations can program your mind into believing them. It's common for athletes and other people who achieve new things to use the idea of repeating affirmations and picturing themselves succeed to change mindset.

Take a minute before each pool session to think or say to yourself some affirmations, maybe as you're on the way to the pool in the car, changing into your swimsuit or stepping in the pool. You can use affirmations as you close out or open your day, and as you reflect on the things you've tried and accomplished.

"I find such healing at the ocean – it goes from the deepest exhale ever when I get there to the most renewed energy by the time I leave."

~ Pattie Cornute, Founder of Lipedema Fitness ~

Sample Affirmations Related to Aqua therapy
- All I must do is make a bit of progress today. It doesn't have to be perfect.
- All movement, and any time in the water is so much better than being in the bed or on the couch.
- Deep breathing exercise in the water is so cleansing. I love it.
- I am building myself a stronger and better body today.
- I am strong in the water.
- I am thankful for my health.
- I can't wait to dance in the water.
- I feel confident in this swimsuit because it provides good support and coverage. I'm so glad I feel confident and can go in public. Thank you to the fashion industry for designing a suit that makes women love them.
- I feel good in the water.
- I get energy by moving in the water.
- I look forward to kicking my legs and feeling them get stronger.
- I look forward to this time working on myself.
- I love being able to run in the water.
- I move freely in the water.
- I'm fighting hard, and this exercise is known to help lymphedema and lipedema. I'm helping to prevent progression of lymphedema and lipedema.
- I'm helping my swelling go down when I get in the water.
- I'm not afraid.
- I'm proud of myself for getting in the pool.
- I'm taking care of my body doing something fun.
- I'm thankful for the ability to move today.
- Just move. Just move.
- My body is a human body, and I look like a lot of other people on this earth. I am like other people.
- Repetition as I swim: I'm thankful for my healthy body and I'm grateful for what I'm able to do today. Swimming feels good and is so fun and good for me.

- Swimming and dancing in the water is fun. The more I do, the more I enjoy it.
- Swimming gives me joy.
- Water is healing to me and being in it restores me.

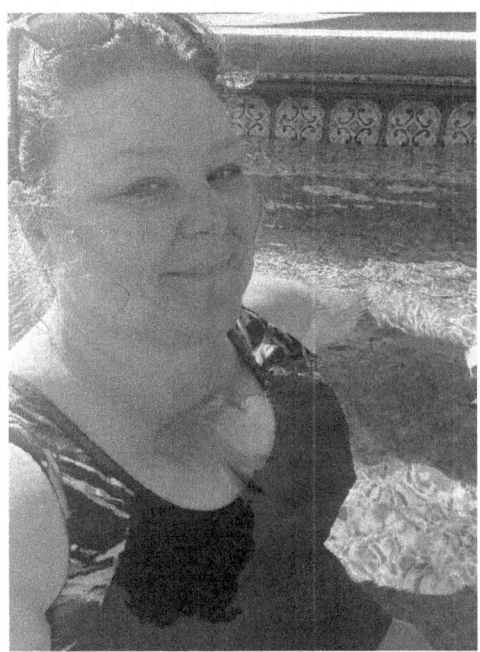

Ohmmmmm!

Your Own Meaningful Affirmations

What other things can you, or do you say to yourself as an affirmation to remember that the exercise you're doing is wonderful? What else can you think of that when you repeat enough with movement, will become your truth, that would be helpful to live on in your mind?

- Add your own ideas here:

  _____

- Add your own ideas here:

  _____

- Add your own ideas here:

  _____

- Add your own ideas here:

  _____

Progress, Not Perfection!

Any movement is better than staying on the couch or the bed. No one cares what you do in the water, and honestly, no one is watching you or grading you on your sweet dance moves, how flexible you are or if you keep time with the instructor and the music. Everything in the water is for you, and only you, so make the best of it. If you're in a class and not kicking as high as the others in the room, who cares and so what? Move when it feels good and stop when you're done. If you're doing one thing more than you did yesterday, you're doing good. Aim for progress, not perfection and enjoy the freedom of being able to move in the water.

"When the water is calm, take as much distance as possible with your boat!"

~ Mehmet Murat İldan ~

Where and When to Swim

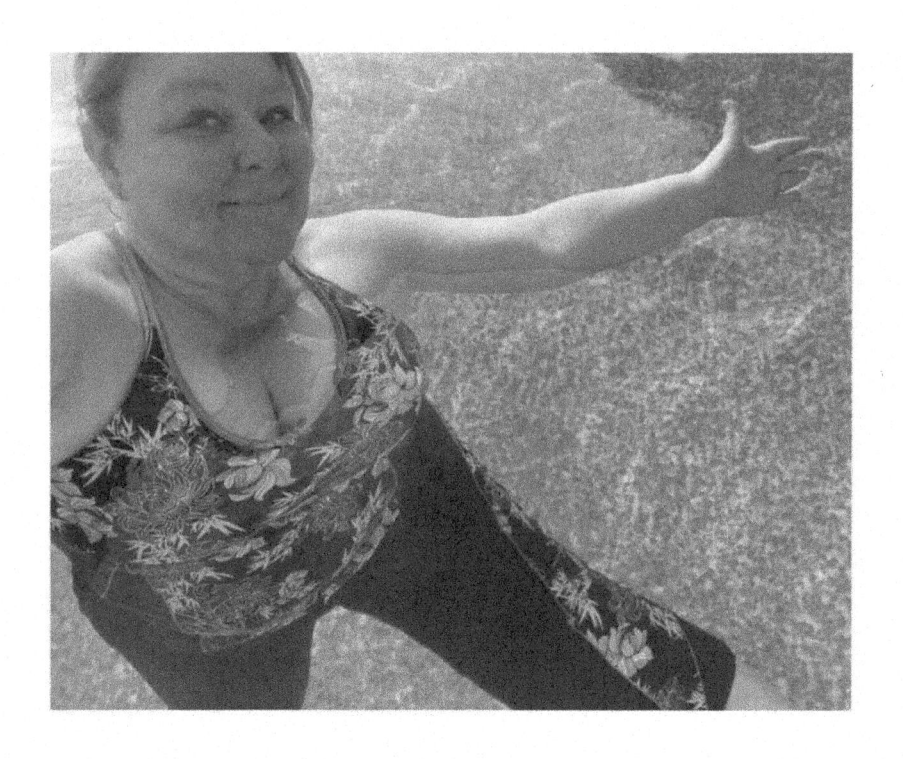

Chapter 5: Where and When to Swim

The good news about choosing aqua therapy to help your lipedema and lymphedema is that all you really need is a body of water. The depth of pool is based on your preference and pools available: deep water is great, but shallow pools also are so helpful, especially for non-swimmers. Remember ALL that compression you're getting at just three feet deep – more than compression garments.

Here are a few tips to make your aqua therapy experience more pleasant:

Choose a facility with a pool that is heated, with temperatures around 30-34° C (86-93°F), to help your muscles and connective tissues relax. Cold water can be painful for those of us with damaged joints, and water that is 94°F or hotter is not recommended for patients with lymphedema and lipedema as hot water can worsen swelling and damage tissues.

Get to know the pool you're using. There are usually lap times, and water times, and my local Y even has water exercise times and you just kind of grab a spot in the pool. What I *do* avoid is the dreaded Family Swim Time in public pools– a guaranteed time of no peace and quiet, curious onlookers or aggravating water wars.

WARNING: Some folks may find that flareups of inflammation are triggered by being in chlorine or bromine pools and may have to find a salt or freshwater alternative. Another alternative is to find an outdoor pool because the chemicals aren't so saturated in the air.

Where to Find "Your" Water

- You may be able to find facilities that lead classes especially designed for lymphedema (lipedema specific is hard to find, so just go to the lymphedema classes).
- Look for professionals, such as certified aquatic therapists, physical therapists or physiotherapists experienced with lymphedema or lipedema treatments, who can develop an exercise program tailored to your specific needs. Some hospitals have physiotherapists and therapy pools with special training who

can show you how to do the exercises and adjust them to help with your range of motion or specific goals.
- Local colleges may have swim classes. Even local high schools might have pools with public hours.
- The local neighborhood association pool.
- Gyms with indoor or outdoor pools.
- Hotel pools and apartment complexes. You might even be able to pay for a day pass at either.
- The ocean and lakes.
- Senior center pools.
- Finally, your home, or a friend's home, pool!

Speaking of a home pool, here are a couple of ideas that might help you if you're really thinking about putting a pool in:

Could a Prescription for Swimming Help?

According to the Centers for Disease Control and Prevention, swimming provides a cardiovascular workout that promotes heart and lung health, improves strength and flexibility, increases stamina, and improves balance and posture. Swimming puts less strain on joints and connective tissues than other forms of exercise. If you're planning to cover the costs of your home pool, ask your doctor for a prescription for swimming or aquatic therapy.

You Might Qualify for a Tax Deduction for an at-Home Pool

In some cases, you can deduct a swimming pool on your US taxes. This includes the installation costs for the year you install the pool and then operating, cleaning, and maintenance costs. The pool has to be entirely used for your medical exercise, and there are other rules, like that your doctor needs to prescribe swimming or aquatic therapy for your health condition, so this is something to consider. Definitely talk to your tax person before doing this and refer to IRS rules (currently publication 502 on medical and dental expenses), or the rules of your local country before making the decision to put in a pool. If you're outside the US, look into your local tax code to see if there might be a benefit as well!

When to Swim

The time of day you choose to swim is entirely up to you.

Some of us like a quiet start to the day, while I've lately enjoyed swimming late in these hot Oklahoma summer evenings. My treat is that after I'm done exercising, I float on my back and talk to the heavens while I'm looking at the stars.

A great time to swim is after travelling, or anytime you're swollen up or having a flare. Water compression can really help ease the pain and reduce swelling very quickly. If you're tempted to lie in bed when you're swollen, remember, "motion is lotion." And movement really helps.

A common schedule idea is to try to swim 3 time a week or more. But any time is better than nothing. In fact, any time you're not sitting, laying down or otherwise being immobile is certainly better than doing those things.

How Long to Swim in Each Session

This is a question with many answers. Several people on the online support groups swear by staying at least 45 minutes per session. I personally committed to being in the water and vertical (for best compression) at least 30 minutes, with movement of any type at least 20 of those on days when it's cold, and longer when the weather is nice. Some people enjoy a swim for as long as two hours a session and believe that they get the most benefit when they stay longer. You be the judge by watching your swelling and seeing how much time it takes to get some fluid up and out.

For the purposes of getting started you will need to start slowly. Maybe a five-minute water walk is what will help you for the first few weeks, and you can add on some other exercises as you build up endurance. Do not feel pressure to go for a long time all at once. Remember swimming work is hard and when you get out of the pool, you're going to feel more tired than if you'd walked on land. So, take it easy on yourself and build up to your target time gradually. It's OK! Anything we do more than sitting on the couch is a great move.

How Often to Perform Aqua therapy

Schedule regular aqua therapy sessions on your calendar at least two to three times a week, for best results. Of course, if you want to do more, do more, just don't overdo it by expending too much energy and causing unbridled fatigue.

Try to stick with swimming for a couple of months before deciding to move on to another exercise. You'll find the longer you stay, the more you're getting stronger and more flexible, and are able to keep swelling under control.

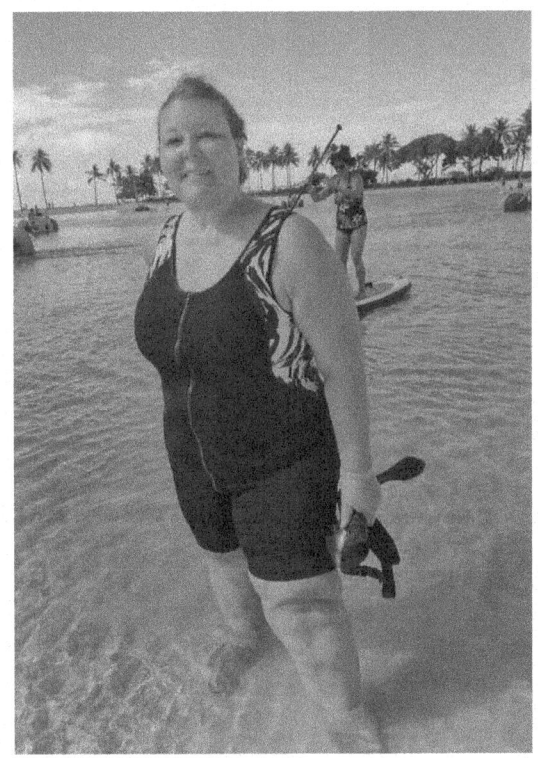

I love the water, so much.

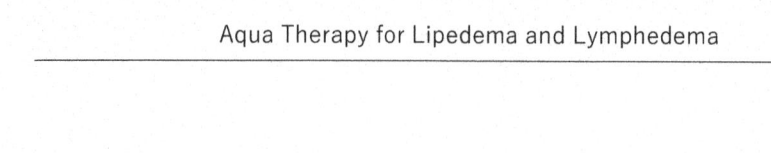

"A river doesn't just carry water, it carries life."

~ Ahmit Kalantri ~

Supplies

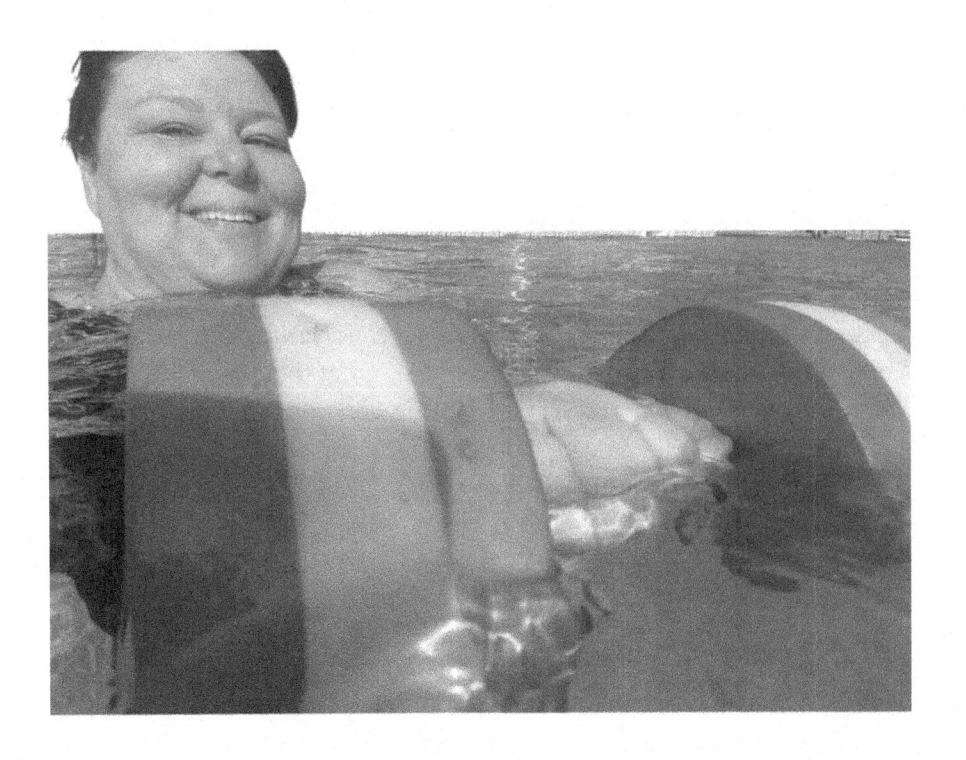

Chapter 6: Supplies

All you need is a pool or a natural body of water and you're good to go! What's so great is that if you have no supplies, you can get the job done anywhere in the world with water. Of course, there are things you can buy to enhance your swim, but it is not needed to get started. Don't let supplies hold you back.

What to Wear

You don't need anything special. Don't feel like you even have to wear a bathing suit. As long as your outfit has been washed and dried, making its dye set, doesn't have a lot of metal, strings from cutting off jeans or anything pokey on it, you should be fine. You can even get in the water wearing leggings and a t-shirt. I see this shorts-or-leggings-with-a-t-shirt look in the pool, on women and men, every time I go to a water class at the YMCA. I mean it, every time.

Another thing to consider is that many folks get in the pool waist or chest deep and are able to keep from having to get their hair wet or lose their makeup for the day. It is very possible to do water exercise without having to spend hours getting ready for the day a second time afterwards.

FAQ: Do I wear compression in the water?
No, I don't, and I personally don't recommend that you do, unless it's for cosmetic needs or personal choice. The water provides the compression, so you don't need it (see my chapter on Water as Nature's Compression). Enjoy that free time away from all the not-so-great things wearing compression brings as a treat for doing your workout. It's so wonderful! In-water sports are the only type of exercise that should be done without compression, literally because you're already getting compression by being in the water. For lipedema and lymphedema patients, everything else exercise-wise on dry land should be done while wearing compression.

TIP: Remember to put your compression garments back on as soon as you can after exiting the water and rinsing off. This will allow the limb reduction you've just achieved by being in the water and moving to stay reduced as long as possible. Talk to your doctor on this.

TIP: Lotions, oils and other chemicals can alter the lifespan of your compression, so I recommend using lotion after you remove compression at bedtime (not immediately after your aqua therapy, unless you're heading straight to bed) for both optimal skin care and the longevity of your compression.

Answer to a Frequently Asked Question? Where Do I get My Aquatard type swimming suits?
Every time I go in public with these one piece suits on, I get the question, so here's my answer. I get them from a small business called JunoActive ® that is an online plus size swim and activewear company. I love what this company makes and the quality of their products, so I chose to do affiliate marketing for them on the LegsLikeMine.com presence. Here's a link to their site:

QR Link to JUunoactive.com

Confidence in a Swimming Suit

- Wear a suit that covers what you don't want to highlight (like an aquatard, skirt or swim capris) or that has a feature to draw the eye up, like a V-Neck. I personally normally wear aquatards that go to my knees in public. Whoever invented those is my hero, because it changed how I enjoy the water in public forever.
- At home, I wear what I want, including (gasp!) a bikini, because the water and sun feel good on my belly that doesn't see the light of day too often. Owning a bikini has changed my confidence, too.
- You can come to class in your suit with a dress over it, literally take it off as you're stepping in the water and throw it right back on afterwards to go home. No one says you have to use the locker room! I always show up in my suit with a dress on top of it to save time, and I whisk my dress off in the shower room right before I get in the pool. I'm just not a "getting naked in front of other people" kind of person anyway.
- Swim with the senior citizens even if you aren't one. I do! I love the vibe of seniors who aren't in a hurry, their classes are at my fitness level, and they have proven to be very body positive and real in all my experiences taking many water fitness classes. I usually get questions about where I buy my swimming outfits from, in fact, during these classes.
- Exercise and wearing a swimsuit may be intimidating for you, and I validate that. In the water, there's no one to judge your form or how fast or high you're moving your body, and the water doesn't care. No one is watching your legs jiggle. In fact, when I'm at the beach, I often tell myself, "I'm never seeing these people again. I'm having fun!"
- Try coming to the water 2-3 days a week. It's hard walking out in that bathing suit the first time, yes for me too. But the more you go, the more confident you'll become. Get a suit you love that covers you the way you want to be covered.
- Remember your physical body language can literally change your brain, so walk to the pool with shoulders back, chin up and walk

Aqua Therapy for Lipedema and Lymphedema

with purpose. Tell your body you are confident by the way you stand, and you will believe it.
- Smile while you're working out because it really does tell your brain that you're having fun.
- Having a successful session will build up confidence for future sessions, so do what you can and gain confidence with each time you visit the pool.

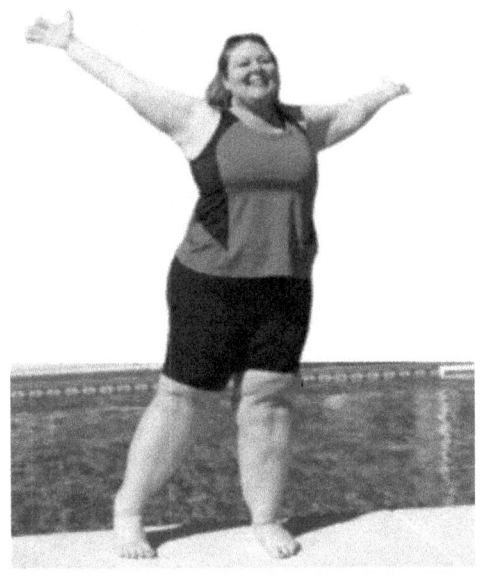

Feeling confident in my swimsuit makes all the difference.

Caring for your Swimsuit

Specialty swimsuits like the aquatards or tankini sets I wear can be expensive, often more than $150 each, and they are worth it. And mine often last more than several seasons without wear because I care for them well. Here are my tips:

- Treat a quality suit just like a compression garment. Treat a cheap suit like fancy lingerie.
- It will begin to stretch out after around 12 hours of wear. Regular washing will help retain the elastic properties.
- Machine or hand wash using a mild soap or detergent (no chorine, fabric softener or bleach).

- In the washer use a mesh lingerie bag, the gentle cycle and cool water. Don't over agitate or stretch and don't wring suits.
- Squeeze out excess water and roll the suit in a towel to remove extra water.
- Check your local gym to see if they have a little bathing suit water extractor machine. They're usually near the locker room showers. I rinse mine out in the shower and extract the water from the suit, keeping it from getting mildewy or stinky before I wash it next. TIP: If you do use an extractor, make sure to put all the zippers, doo dads, and buttons in the bottom so they don't get caught.
- Always air-dry swimsuits, as extra heat can weaken the elastic.

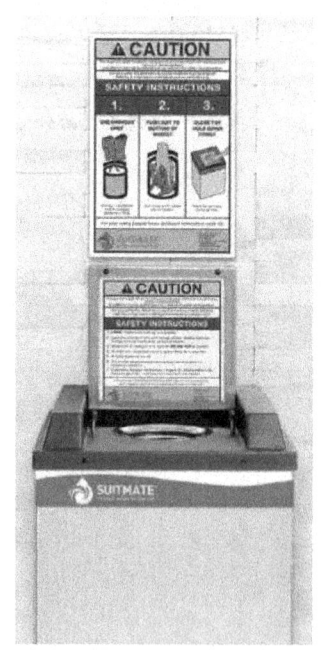

Swimsuit Water Extractor at my Local YMCA.

Other Supplies You Might Be Interested In

There are all kinds of little floatie things that you can use to aid in your aqua therapy. From dumbbells, to floating pillows, check online at places like Amazon to see more than you'd ever need. Remember though, you really don't have to have anything to get started. Here are some ideas:

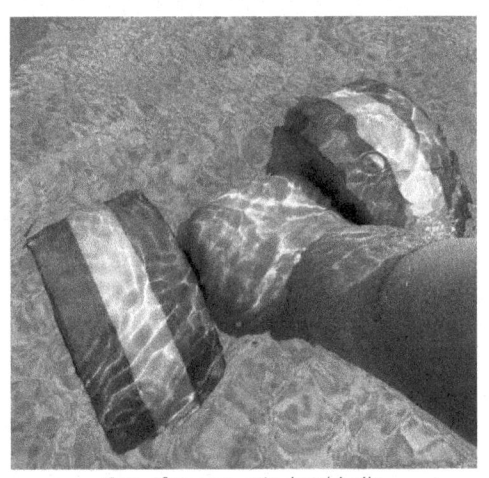

One of my aquatic dumbbells.

- Aquatic Dumbbells: Use these when you need a little bit of extra flotation to hold in your hands when doing flutter kicks, or to place under your armpits when bicycling. These are also fabulous for a simple way to add resistance when doing arm exercises, or to moves like jumping jacks and cross-country skiing in the water.
- Ear Plugs: If you have any issues with getting water in your ears, keep a pair in your swim bag handy. There are many days now that I get my whole swim in without getting my hair or ears wet, but it's nice to have them, just in case.
- Flotation Belt or Life Jacket: Great for non-swimmers and for deep water exercise.
- Hair Ties: If you have long hair, pull it up quickly and keep it dry.
- Kickboards: Great for doing some of the exercises I list here, keeping in the pool as a quick safety grab, and for floating on after a good workout.

- Pool Noodles: Really such an inexpensive little tool that can be replaced easily if lost. I use these to float on for bicycles and other extension exercises, but also for exercises where I push my legs and feet on them (see the car clutch exercises in the book).

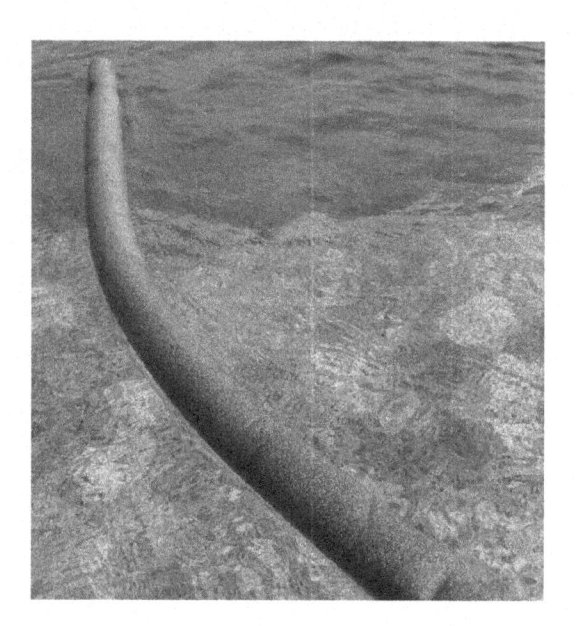

  -

- Sunscreen, Sunglasses and Hat: If you're swimming outside.
- Swim Goggles: If you like doing strokes that get your face wet.
- Swimmers Ear Drops: Great if you're swimming in a natural body of water to dry the water out and kill any little bacteria that may have gotten in.
- Towel: Most gyms will have smallish sized towels available. I usually bring my own, large enough to wrap around me as needed.
- Water Bottle: It's important to stay hydrated while doing water activities. We don't realize how much we're sweating I the water, but remember to take drinks as you go, and before your aqua therapy session.

- Water Gloves: These are webbed between the fingers to provide increased resistance in water during water exercise. Open fingers help maintain a feel for the water. I personally do not use them because I cup my hands for resistance, but there are ladies in my classes that swear by them.

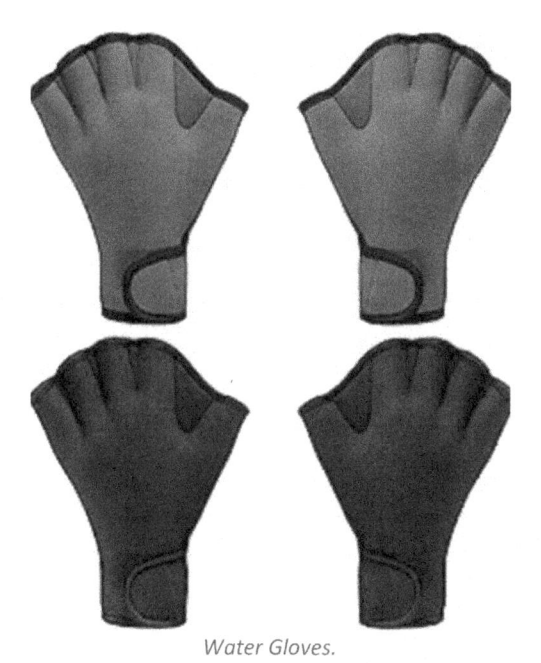

Water Gloves.

- Water Shoes: If you're swimming in any place where your feet can get cut or scratched (this includes pools with a scratchy bottom during water aerobics, especially), wear water shoes or even old tennis shoes to protect them.
- Water Weights: A pound of extra weight makes a tremendous difference when you're doing your leg workouts. I'd start without them because the added resistance in water will be a huge difference to land-based exercise anyway. But maybe someday? Who knows!

"Water is the soul of the earth."

~ W.H. Auden ~

Aqua Therapy for Lipedema and Lymphedema

Safety

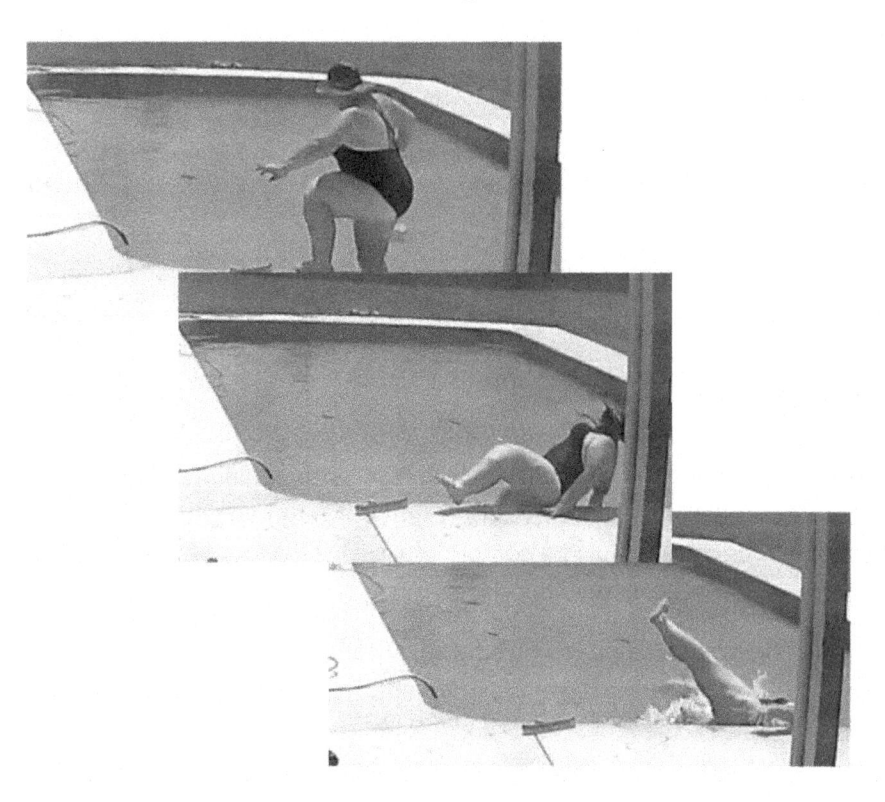

Chapter 7: Safety

Yep. That's me in the pictures on the previous page, slipping right into the pool. And it's not a staged picture. PS I didn't get hurt, thankfully.

Obviously, swimming only helps your lipedema and lymphedema, if you survive it! The pictures on the page before this are real pics from our home security camera, the first day our pool was ready to swim in. And, it didn't have handrails installed yet. I learned the hard way that I must take it a little slower and use safety equipment. We immediately installed a heavy-duty handrail and slip resistant grips on the steps after I discovered how slippery the steps really were. Now that we've got that story out of the way...

Safety for Non-Swimmers

You don't have to be able to swim to benefit from aqua therapy. You can do many exercises, especially walking, in shallow water up to chest height, so exercise at a depth that is comfortable and safe for you.

You can also use floats at any time. Go as deep as you are comfortable, but anything deeper than the waist will give you the most benefit.

Non-swimmers should not do any form of aquatic exercise alone. So have a partner or attend a class. It's great to have someone near to help you if you slip or even accidentally make your way into the deep end.

STOP! Contraindications for Aqua therapy

If you have any of these conditions, don't swim or get in the water. Talk to your doctor and have a supervisor present only after you get the go ahead from your doctor. This isn't a comprehensive list, so always talk with your doctor before starting a swim program.

- Being sick in general (like having a cold, the flu, or COVID). Therapy and exercise are not helpful if your body is trying to heal. It needs to focus, and you won't get the benefits if you try to work out when you're sick. Let your lymphatic system take care of

getting rid of the crud and not extra stuff you're stirring up with new movement.
- Catheters and Ostomies
- Chlorine Allergy
- Fear of water
- Fever
- Heart disease
- Incontinence/Diarrhea
- Infections
- Kidney Diseases
- Open wounds
- Perforated Ear Drums
- Recent Chemotherapy or Radiation
- Recent Surgery
- Severe Epilepsy
- Skin conditions
- Tracheotomy
- Urinary Tract Infection

Fatigue

Swimming and water exercise bring about much more resistance than we're used to. It's really easy to feel so great that we overdo it. Take it easy because when you get out of the pool, you're going to be tired. And you also don't want to cause injury or encourage swelling by doing too much exercise or too high intensity exercise due to the wonderful gravity defying feeling we get in the water.

Watch for your level of fatigue after your sessions. You may notice you're more tired than normal, which is a sign that your next aqua therapy session could be made shorter or easier to get you through the rest of your day.

Finally, please let your doctor know you're planning to start some water exercise. They may even have ideas for the best exercises to help you, and based on your particular medical situation, exercises they recommend you avoid.

Water Temperature

Note: This book's benefits are for swimming in a pool, not a hot tub. While some folks with lipedema and lymphedema self-report good experiences of using a hot tub, I am not recommending that. Using hot tubs can make your legs or arms swell up. This is because direct heat causes capillaries in the skin to dilate, and could cause an increase in the interstitial fluid, making edema worse or even trigger previously nonexistent lymphedema. So, talk with your doctor before using a hot tub, and perform the exercises in this book in a pool that's in the temperature range I mention below, just to be safe.

Warm water feels great if you have sore joints, aching muscles, etc. For me personally, very cold water makes my joints hurt, so I avoid it. Research written by D. Tidhar, who created a group exercise program for lymphedema patients called Aqua Lymphatic Therapy, discussed temperature in depth in some of her papers. Their recommendation is that water temperature from 78.8 to 91.4° F is safe for slow limb movement without causing additional swelling.

Other research papers I've reviewed noted that water up to 94 degrees is safe for patients with lipedema and lymphedema. So being in water that ranges from that 91.4 to 94-degree mark is good for folks who are literally standing in the water just for the compression but not necessarily the active exercise component. Other aquatic therapy programs recommend similar temperature ranges as well. Something to think about if you have control over the temperature of your own pool at home. I prefer 84-85 degrees, although keeping my pool warm in the winter is expensive!

Cleanliness

Make sure you're swimming in clean water. We with lipedema and lymphedema are sensitive to things that may not bother unaffected people, so we need to be really careful about not ingesting water or allowing any wounds to come in contact with water.

I hate this because the lakes where I am are brown – you cannot see through them, and I've basically stopped getting in these bodies of water because I don't want to get an infection. I still swim in the ocean in areas where the water is clear and the water is not stagnant, if I have no open wounds or skin issues going on.

Hypermobility and Swimming

Many, but not all, people who have lipedema also suffer from joint hypermobility (you may hear it referred to as Hypermobile Ehlers-Danlos Syndrome or hEDS) because they are both loose connective tissue disorders and are somewhat related (not all the research is done on this yet). To oversimplify hEDS, its symptoms include being really flexible ("double jointed") and have pain because you can overextend and even subluxate/dislocate joints, often unintentionally. There are other symptoms as well. A formal diagnosis of hEDS has several criteria (no blood test yet) that you can find at the Ehlers-Danlos Society's website. Regardless of having a diagnosis or not, hypermobility can cause injury and it's something to be cautious about when you're swimming. I personally avoid several swimming strokes and moves because they cause my knees to subluxate, and it hurts bad at the time, and then for a couple of days afterwards when I get a 'good one.'

QR Link to the Ehlers-Danlos Society's Diagnostic Criteria for Hypermobile Ehlers Danlos Syndrome.

Whether you have hEDS formally or undiagnosed or don't have it at all (be thankful!), one of the things you can do to protect joints is to avoid overextending or putting stress on them on purpose. This can make any exercise an interesting challenge and it's something to pay attention to in the pool as well.

Strokes like the breaststroke involve a sudden kick of both legs and can cause a lot of harsh movement on the knees and for me, cause me to subluxate (I call it my "knees flipping inside out"), so I avoid them. In fact, although I'm no doctor, I've felt enough pain from trying the breaststroke that I just recommend avoiding the breaststroke for lipedema in general. A ton of swimmers who are breaststroke specialists have knee problems, so why even go there. I also occasionally struggle with sidekicks and dislocate then, but not a full on lock up like I do with the breaststroke.

There are so many exercises you can do in the water that strengthen supporting muscles, that water exercise can help to keep your mobility when you are hypermobile. This is an area to talk to a physical therapist about if you're having trouble finding the right exercise. Also, there are numerous swimmers' knee braces even on Amazon (I'm not sure how many will fit very large legs, but it's worth a look if you're really dedicated to doing the breaststroke in the water).

For this reason, I removed a lot of exercises from my own routine and from the book. So, you won't see a lot of jumping or jerky movements in this book but there is so much we can do safely.

The other thing to pay attention to if you're hypermobile is over stretching. Stretching carefully can help you be more aware of your body movements and how to control them. But, as you start swimming, if you are working with one of your hypermobile locations, consider skipping any stretching exercises so you do not overstress the joint, or make the hypermobility worse. There is information on the internet that contradicts each other regarding stretching with hypermobility so be careful and ask your physical therapist for advice on how to stretch safely.

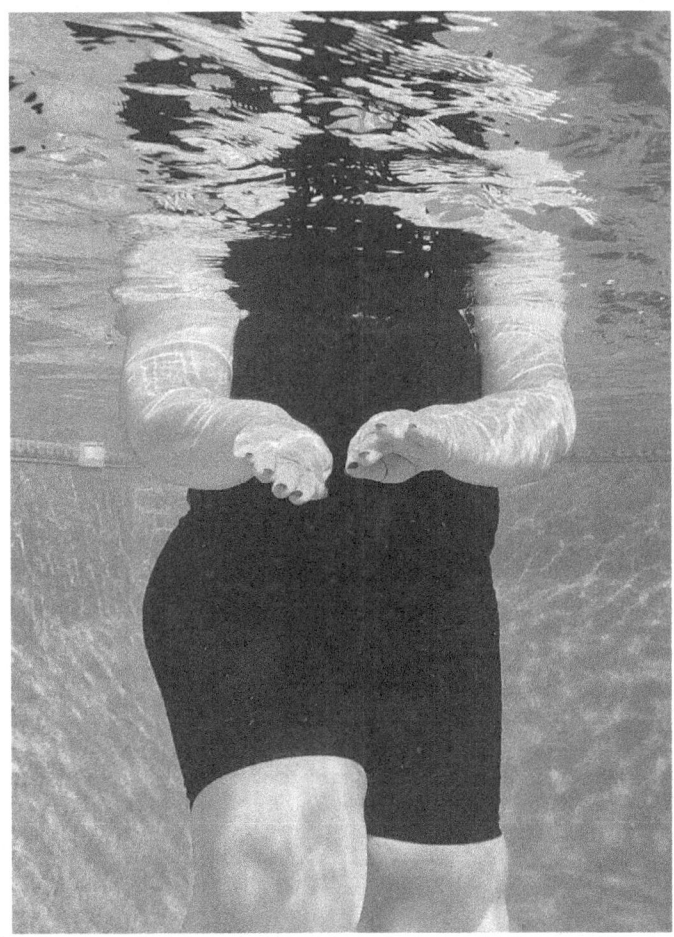

A walking breaststroke is better on the joints of people with hypermobility because it avoids the sudden kicks of a traditional breaststroke.

Don't Overdo It! And Other Random Safety Tips

- Start slowly and build up your session's duration over time. Maybe try for fifteen minutes in the water at first, or five. I know I've said this already, but that means it's important and real.
- Keep standard safety equipment where it should be.
- Put a floatation device in the water with you so you can grab on while doing exercise or if you're a non-swimmer, lose your footing out of the shallow end.
- Wear a life jacket or flotation belt if you need it. There's no glory in drowning during an aqua therapy session.
- Even if class isn't over, if you're too tired, slow down or stop. If you go to the side to get a drink, and take a little pause, that's fine too. Your instructor knows to watch for signs of fatigue and will understand, I promise. Some classes or routine ideas may be too long for what you're ready for now, and that is totally OK.
- Before going in the water, first check your skin to make sure you have no open wounds, weeping, or skin that is so tight it might rupture. If your skin is getting dried out, use lotion or your creams after you remove compression each night, so you stay moisturized but don't damage your compression during wear.
- If you have any infections of the skin including cellulitis, skip the swim until it's better.
- Don't swim if you're too tired, not feeling well, or are too full.
- Don't do things in the water that hurt. Literally, if it causes pain, stop.
- Pay attention to beach safety and heed the guidance of lifeguards concerning undertow, rocks, etc.
- Wear appropriate footwear, especially in natural or slippery areas.
- Make sure you've let someone know where you are, especially if you're in your backyard pool or plan to be alone, which we don't recommend.
- Don't swim or exercise in a water depth that you're not comfortable in.

- Make sure you have a safe way into a pool. Install arm rails, chair lifts, and yes, slip resistance on the steps, etc.
- Keep a cell phone handy.
- Overexercising with a lymphatic system challenge can be harmful to your tissues by building up too much lactic acid that may not flow out normally. If you "feel the burn," consider backing off the amount of strain on your body by reducing intensity or the duration of the exercise. .

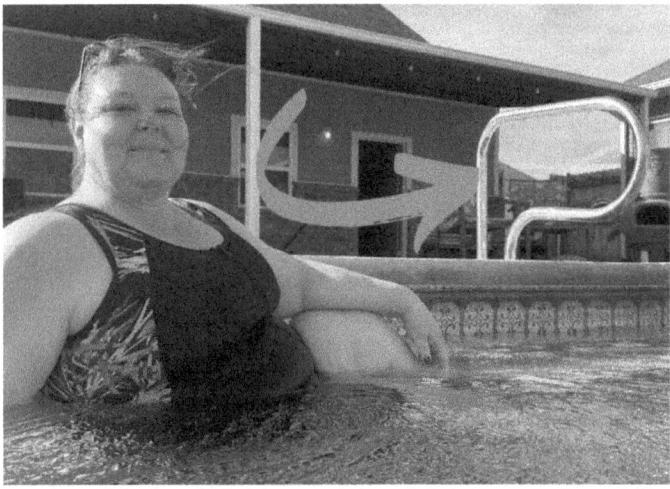

Image of the handrails in my pool, especially important since I fell!

Individually, we are one drop. Together we are an ocean.

~ Ryunosuke Satoro ~

Aqua Therapy Basics

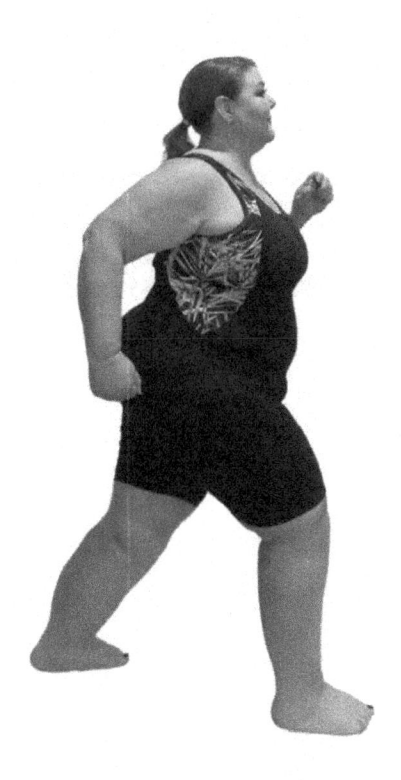

Chapter 8: Aqua therapy Basics

*Note: I have a playlist on **my YouTube channel** that is dedicated to all things Aqua therapy for Lipedema and Lymphedema. There are videos of exercises, tips, and chats from the pool to enjoy and learn as I continue to learn more about aqua therapy and deepen my own practice.*

Please scan this code to go straight to my channel's playlist. If you have questions about how I do any of the exercises, drop me a line at LegsLikeMine@gmail.com, and I'll be happy to show you on my channel.

QR Link to my LegsLikeMine YouTube channel: www.YouTube.com/c/LegsLikeMine.

General Tips on Exercising in the Water

Consult your doctor before starting any new exercise program, including aqua therapy, to ensure that it is safe and appropriate for you.

1. Begin with gentle exercises: Starting your aqua therapy routine with gentle exercises and stretches is essential to prevent any strain or injury. Begin by walking in the pool or performing simple stretches, such as ankle rotations or shoulder rolls.
2. Gradually increase intensity and duration: As you become more comfortable with the exercises, gradually increase the intensity and duration of your aqua therapy routine. This can include adding resistance training, increasing the speed or distance of your walk, or incorporating interval training.
3. Use flotation devices: Flotation devices can be useful to help support your weight and reduce the risk of any injury. Using water weights, kickboards, or pool noodles can also add resistance to your exercises and increase the intensity of your workout.
4. Focus on lymphatic drainage: Aqua therapy is an excellent way to stimulate lymphatic drainage and reduce swelling associated with lipedema. Gentle movements, such as leg lifts, foot circles, and flutter kicks, can help improve lymphatic flow and reduce fluid buildup.
5. Stay hydrated: It's essential to stay hydrated during aqua therapy sessions, as you'll be losing fluids through sweat and exercise. Be sure to drink plenty of water before, during, and after your workout to prevent dehydration and maintain energy levels.

Breathing

IMPORTANT! Every aqua therapy session in the pool should start and end with some deep breathing to help you relax and focus, and to move lymphatic fluid. When our diaphragm moves up and down with deep abdominal breathing, it helps return lymphatic fluid to the blood stream by opening up our lymph nodes. Think about breathing while you exercise to Include regulated, controlled breathing to help intentionally clear up and move lymph fluid.

If you've been swimming for your condition before, but skipping the deep breathing before and after, adding this simple step will increase the value of your time in the water.

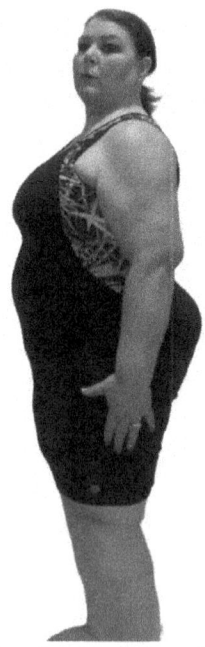

Side view of what my belly looks like when I'm doing a deep abdominal breath. Pushed out and full of air.

Simple Deep Abdominal Breathing

At the start of your session, do this in the pool in waist deep or deeper water three times: Anytime you're in the water, practice these exercises a few times, but especially before and after an exercise session.

1. From a kneeling or standing position, place your hands on your belly.
2. Inhale deeply through your nose while breathing in enough to make your belly push out (think about how your hands feel when you breathe against them on your belly). Hold the breath for four seconds.
3. Slowly exhale through your mouth.
4. Repeat this, but now push the breath out fast and hard until you cannot squeeze any more air out. Deep, slow breath in to fill the belly, then hard, fast push up from the diaphragm to exhale everything. Do this three times or more.

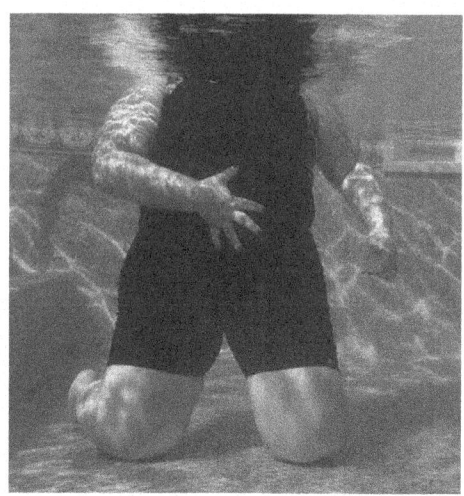

How I do simple deep abdominal breathing with my hand on my belly to feel the air as I inhale, hold, and exhale. This can be done from a kneeling or standing position.

Take a Lymphatic Break!

IMPORTANT! After completing your deep breathing, take a minute to open up your lymphatics for good flow. Regardless of what water exercises I select for my session, I will start and finish all sessions with breathing, and simple lymphatic self-massage.

Simple Abdominal Massage

All lymphatic self-massage (manual lymphatic drainage, MLD) can start in the abdomen area. That's where the 'main drain' of the lymphatic is, so it's the best area to clear first, then follow up with any limbs, and then finish back in the abdomen.

There are many ways to do this, but here are a few ways I like to do it in the water.

Place your hands gently on your abdomen (see figure) and just rub in light circles. Sometimes I will do a gentle sweeping up motion on my belly. Five-ten times is enough. (Remember that game where we used to try to pat our heads and rub our bellies at the same time? It's that, only without the head part.)

Another option for simple abdominal massage is to use open hands, starting at the sides of the tummy, and gently stroke in towards the center a few times, as I demonstrate below.

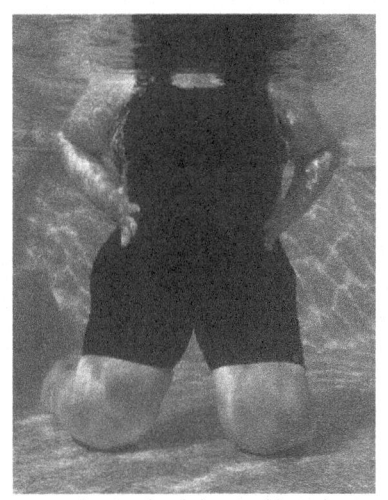

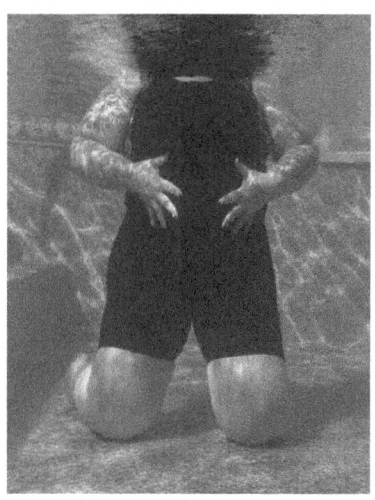

How I do simple abdominal lymphatic massage in the water. This is an open-handed stroke going from the outside of my abdomen, stroking lightly, several times towards the Cisterna Chyli, which is the most common drainage trunk of most of the body's lymphatic system. The stroke ends when my fingers touch. This can be done while standing or kneeling.

Using Water Turbulence to Encourage Lymphatic Flow

A second option for abdominal (or any kind of MLD in the water) is to create turbulence in the water by swiping the water (without touching your body with your hand), up from the groin to the breast area, sweeping the water with it, about ten times. This water turbulence presses on your body and massages the areas it is hitting.

I often make water turbulence with my hands to move water around my legs, chest, armpit and trunk to push the water up on my body, to move the flow in the direction up and out. Here is what it the moves look like when I'm making water turbulence on my abdominal area:

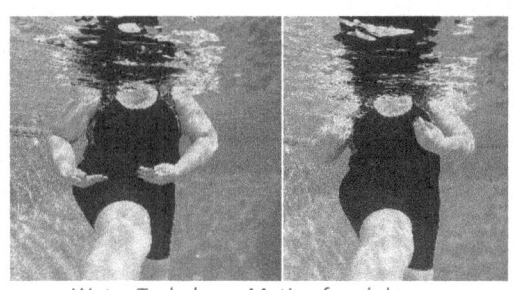

Water Turbulence Motion for abdomen.

Simple Self Leg Manual Lymphatic Drainage (MLD) in the Water

If I'm working on my legs, especially if I'm having a flare or a lot of swelling from travel, I focus on the MLD in these next few steps.

1. Gently press 5-10 times on the crease area between my legs and groin. This activates the superficial inguinal lymph nodes, which is where the lymphatics in the leg drain.
2. Next, I focus on the lymph nodes on the front of my thighs. I press with an open hand in small strokes from the top of my knees to the top of my thighs.
3. Then I like to take an open hand and rub behind my knees five to ten times, gently.

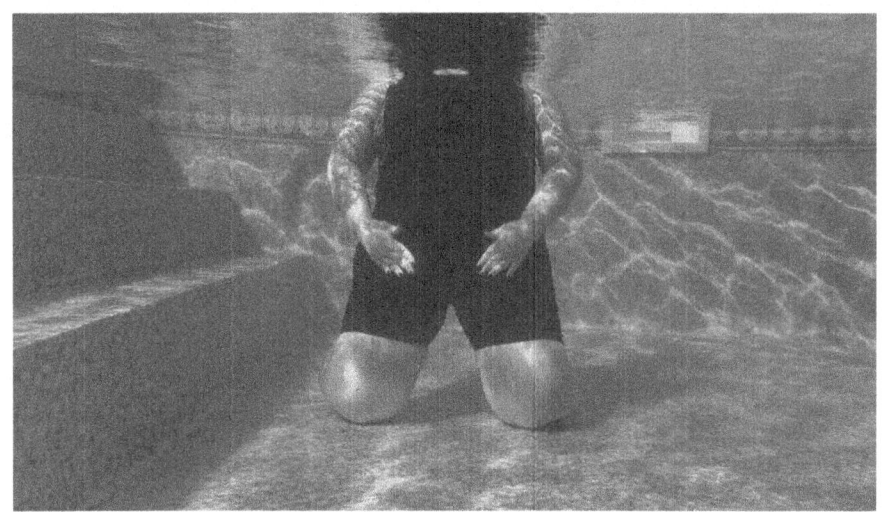

How I do simple groin lymphatic massage in the water. This is an open handed, gentle press on the creased area between the leg and the groin (superficial inguinal lymph node area) five times. It can also involve a light pressing stroke more down towards the medial part of the groin to push fluid down towards the deeper lymph nodes. This can be done while standing or kneeling.

4. Finally, I will place my leg on a stair or shallow floor, and just give it some gentle strokes up to the knee. Note I can kneel in the water. This is something I absolutely wouldn't do on land as kneeling would really hurt my bad knees at this point in my mobility journey! In the water, it's painless.

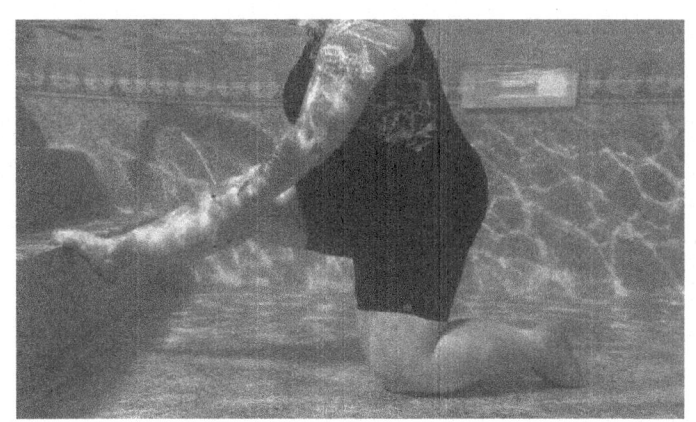

Placing my leg on the pool steps to do some leg MLD up to the groin area.

Another thing I like to do with my legs is when I'm jogging in the water, I will drag my foot up my other leg as it's moving in the jogging motion. This is a natural little lymph boost that I can do while moving the biggest muscles in my body, doubling the impact of the exercise.

Basic Arm MLD in the Water

Arm work can be done as its own workout or in conjunction with leg work. Regardless of this, always start with the abdominal work first because all lymphatics benefit from an open center of the body. Lymphatics flow from out in the arms and legs, towards the center.

1. Starting with the area right above the collarbone and with an open hand, I'll give five to ten light circular motions to activate the lymph nodes there.
2. I move to the armpits and give a gentle five to ten circles there, again with an open, flat hand to be sure I covered the hard-to-feel lymph nodes.
3. I'll continue the light circle work the inside of the elbows five to ten times.
4. Then follow up with a full, sweeping motion up each of the arms. I imagine that I'm literally pushing a circle of fluid up and out as I do this. In extreme cases of edema, you can even sometimes visibly see the bubble of fluid moving when exercises are done slowly.
5. Then I reverse the order. Do armpits, then collarbone area, then stomach again five to ten times.
6. Finish up with some deep breathing.

A lot of lipedema and lymphedema patients already spend time in the water. Adding the deep breathing and self-massage exercises a few times during your session should find you yielding more impressive limb volume reductions in each session. Don't be afraid to experiment with this. Try different light pressures, or rubbing patterns, and more or less repetitions.

Put Your Compression Back On After Your Exercise, Every Time!
IMPORTANT! The benefits of water exercise include all kinds of good things for us, increasing flexibility, stamina, cardiovascular health, mood, and lymphatics. But being in water is proven to reduce swollen limb volume.

Numerous pieces of research show that people with lipedema and lymphedema who perform aquatic therapy will see results in limb volume reduction after as little as one session and the best way to maintain the reduction is to get your compression on immediately after your post-swim shower. If you don't wear compression, the edema reduction will not last as long.

Note: If you don't wear compression (this is true for so many patients, for so many reasons), don't be discouraged from swimming. Getting fluid reduction is a good thing regardless of your compression situation.

Modifying Exercises to Meet You Where You Are

There are many ways to move in the water and many ways you can adjust your effort or motion level to get the workout that feels good for you today. What feels great today may not be enough of a challenge tomorrow, and that's OK. Just adjust your energy level, depth, and amount of motion!

The extra resistance from exercising in water makes you stronger and gives you better endurance with efforts that can be easily changed up. You can control the drag and resistance by using more or less power, changing the depth you're in, making simple hand position changes, or by adding devices like dumbbells to add resistance. Also, the resistance and movement of water, when used right, can even be swooshed in a direction to create turbulence and encourage lymphatic (interstitial) fluid up and out through the body's lymphatic drainage system.

So, we can do exercise in the water at just about any fitness level. Exercise at the level that feels right for you. There are some exercises you prefer to do at one level, while others you may prefer another, and that's great! Remember, if you ever feel pain, stop and do something else or go back to an easier level, smaller motion, or less repetitions. It should feel good!

Very small changes in the way you hold your body, where you are in the pool, and the bigness of your motion make a huge impact in the type of exercise experience you have. The important thing is the be in the water, and to move!

Example Exercise Modifiers for Aquatic Moves

I've made up some charts to show you ways you can modify your movements to make them easier or harder by just making some simple changes. I hope this helps you as your physical fitness and ability to move improve, or if you have something hurt or sore and need to tone it down a bit but want to stay active.

How You Hold Your Hands		
Basic	Cutting the water with your hand	
Intermediate	Using a cupped hand	
Advanced	Using a tool like a floating dumbbell or water gloves.	

	Range of Movement	
Basic	Small motions with lighter pulls and kicks	
Intermediate	Medium effort and middle size motions and medium effort pulls and kicks	
Advanced	High energy, big motions, really pulling and kicking (don't hurt yourself!)	

Depth of Water		
Basic	Working in waist deep water. *Hydrostatic pressure in three feet of water (see p. 55).*	
Intermediate	Working in Chest deep water *Hydrostatic pressure in four feet of water (see p. 54.)*	
Advanced	Working in neck-deep water or water where you don't touch the bottom. *Hydrostatic pressure in five feet of water (see p. 53).*	

	Where You Are in the Pool	
Basic	Working on the side of the pool, doing exercises with half the body while holding on to the side of the pool.	
Intermediate	Working in the shallow end of the pool without hanging on to the pool edge.	
Advanced	Working in the middle of the pool where you use your full body.	

	How Much of Your Body You're Moving	
Basic	Moving one body part at a time, such as standing and doing arm motions for a cross country ski.	
Intermediate	Using arms and legs together to complete a full, big exercise like a cross country ski.	
Advanced	Doing all the body parts at once and adding a toning element, like being in the middle of the pool, and doing a full cross-country ski with arms and legs moving together, using a dumbbell.	

	Resistance	
Basic	Performing an exercise while holding onto a kickboard (that's floating on top of the water) for stability.	
Intermediate	Doing an exercise with just your body.	
Advanced	Doing an exercise with floating dumbbells in your hands.	

Aqua Therapy for Lipedema and Lymphedema

Your Level of Effort and Energy	
Basic	Moving slowly, such as a gentle water walk. If in a class, doing exercises and movements at slower speed than the instructor (yes, it is OK to do this!)
Intermediate	A water jog.
Advanced	Jogging with added resistance under water, using aqua dumbbells.

Water Jogging

"Often, pain prevents many people from tolerating land-based workouts, but these same people can often thrive when utilizing aquatic exercise."

~ LaNese Cummings, Physical Therapist ~

Exercises

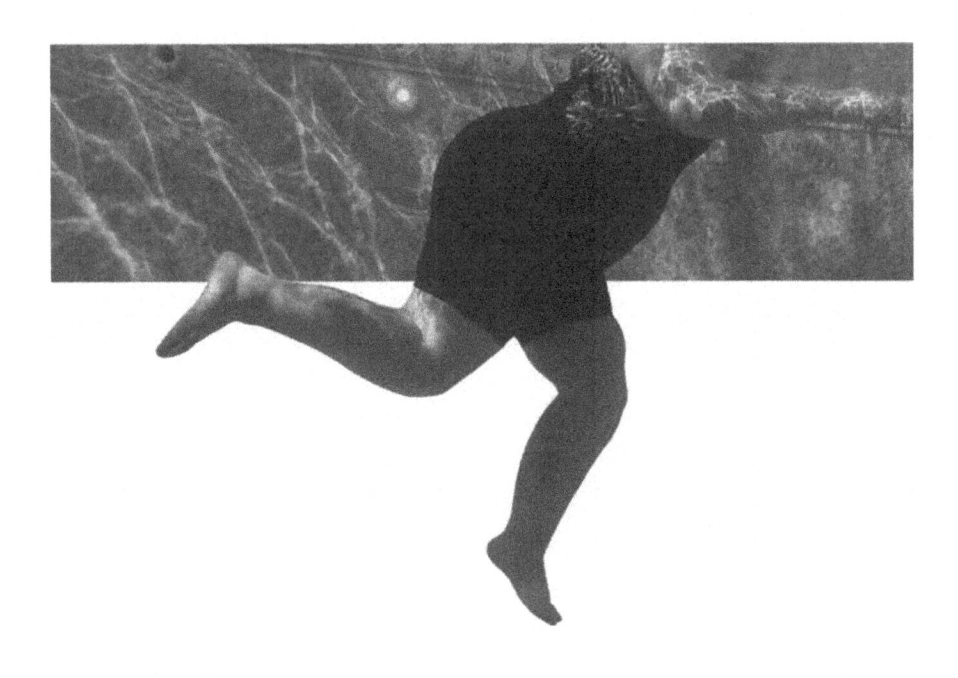

Chapter 9: Exercises

Aqua therapy can be done in formal classes at your local gym or hospital, at home, or at your local community pool. There are a wide range of classes where instructors will walk you through the exercises, and you can enjoy camaraderie with other participants. Even though I've put in a pool, I still attend Water Zumba courses at the YMCA locally just for fun and to learn some new moves. There are also classes like, Water Yoga, Water aerobics, Water Pilates, physical therapy sessions in pools with a trained therapist, Water Arthritis classes, Silver Sneakers and Senior classes (my favorite), along with AquaFit and other branded names, some are designed just for larger people (love this!).

For those of us that have access to a home or community pool, we have the added benefit of proximity to be able to get in and out quicker and do the exercises we need the most on a particular day. We can also control (well, sometimes) the temperature of heated pools to our liking. The exercises I'm going to share with you are ones I personally do.

I specifically pulled out any exercises that involve too much twisting, sudden kicking/thrusting or jumping where we touch the bottom because we have plenty of options without things that could make other conditions (like back issues, or in my case, hypermobile knees that need to be replaced) any worse.

In the following pages, I'll show pictures to help describe many of the exercises, showing a starting and ending point for the movement. There are other exercises where either the picture or narrative might be more self-explanatory, so you won't get the pic and narrative. Please let me know if you have question on any of the exercises or don't find a video on my YouTube channel sharing the exercise. I'll be happy to make one and post it for you. (My channel: www.YouTube.com/c/LegsLikeMine.)

Cardio Exercises

Dance: This may be one of my favorite water exercises. I typically listen to music and depending on what I want out of the water, I put on fun dance music, or soothing bedtime sounds to relax me in a calm swim. But dancing in the water is just the best, because in the water, everyone is a ballerina or a J-Lo.

Walking in the Water: **If you do no other exercise in addition to your breathing and MLD, this is the one to do!**

1. Relax and walk slowly in the water for five to ten minutes, focusing on abdominal breathing. The more relaxed you are, the better it is for your lymphatic system.
2. Feel free to do breaststroke or other arm motions to help propel you as you walk gently. You can even try swinging your arms in the water, or holding dumbbells on the surface as you go about.
3. For additional strength and stability training, try walking sideways and backward.
4. Incorporate arm movements such as swinging or power walking.

Aqua Jogging: This is so much fun because for me, I could NEVER jog on land because the stress is too much for my joints. In the water, I can jog with the best of them.

Here are some tips for aqua jogging: Try to do it without your feet touching the floor. Try to ball up your fists so you're not actually propelling yourself with your hands. And jog! Feel free to use a pool noodle or aqua belt, or even aqua dumbbells under your armpits to help float you. As you progress you can use that same noodle to hold in front of you with one end in each hand. The resistance of the water will add to your workout's impact.

When you're jogging, remember to warm up and cool down and keep the intensity low so you don't overdo it. (See figure.)

Sidestep Walking: **Step to your side with large steps in each direction, using your arms to send water opposite of the direction of your step.**

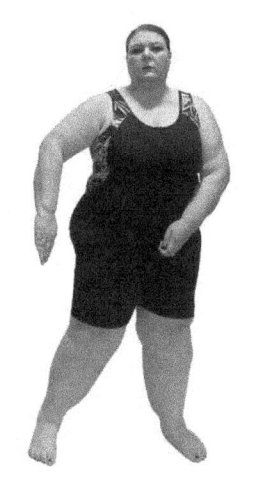

Sidestep walking.

Big Giant Step Walking: **Take the biggest steps you can. Take these slow!**

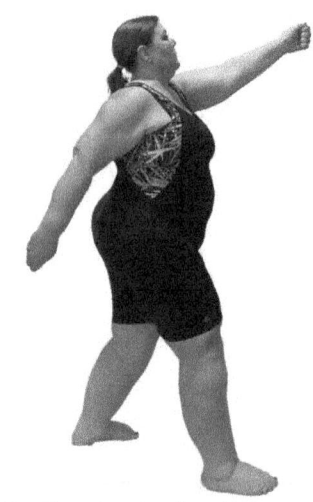

Big, Giant Step Walking!

Running: This can be done in shallower water, or deeper water. The speed is what's important for really getting the heart pumping. You can make it harder by lifting your knees to your chest (or as high as they'll go) while getting the run in.

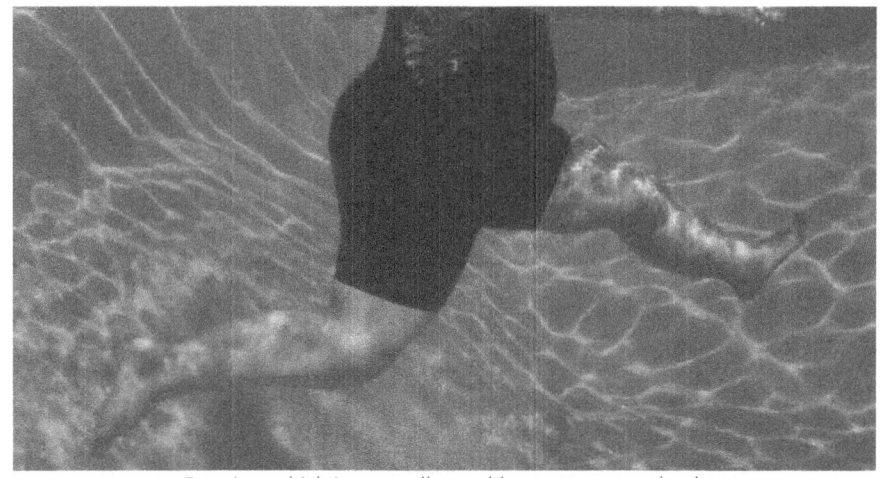

Running, which I personally would not attempt on land.

Treading Water: This is a full body workout, and a move I go to when I'm trying to think up the next exercise I want to perform. Tread in the deep end of the pool, with or without the use of flotation to support you. Move your arms and legs to stay afloat.

Walking with Overhead Arms:

1. Start in waist deep to chest deep water.
2. Move quickly in the water, holding your arms in the air moving them forward and backwards.
3. Also, this is fun to do when you're holding beach balls, dumbbells, or a kickboard, etc. Gets the heart pumping and lymphatics flowing!

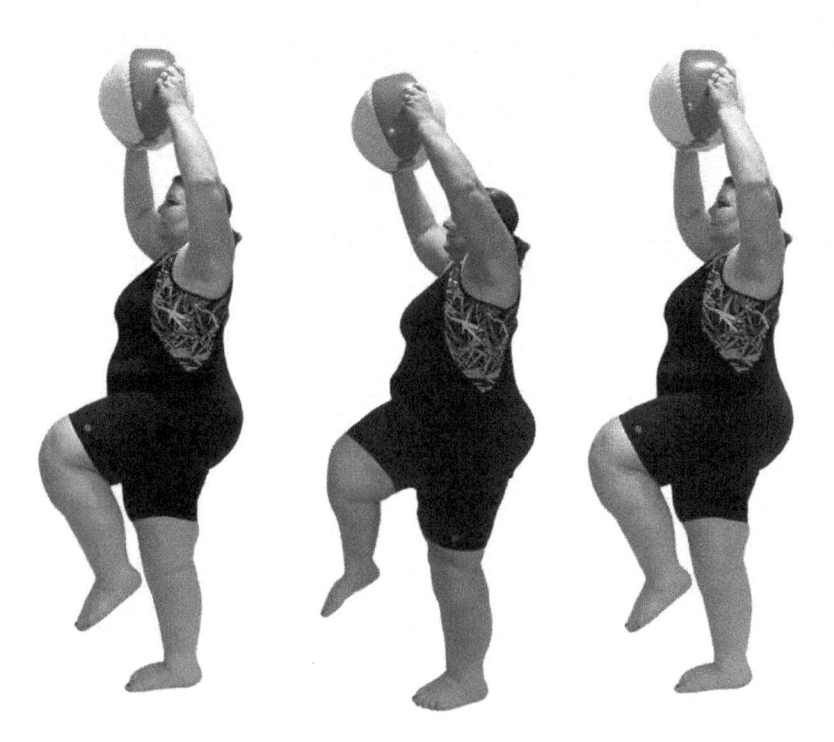

Walking with Overhead Arms.

Deep Water Jumping Jacks: I prefer to do these where my arms only come to the surface, so staying in the deep water isn't a struggle. The most important part for me is that I'm moving my legs and arms out and in repeatedly in controlled motions. Avoid sudden, jerky motions to save your joints!

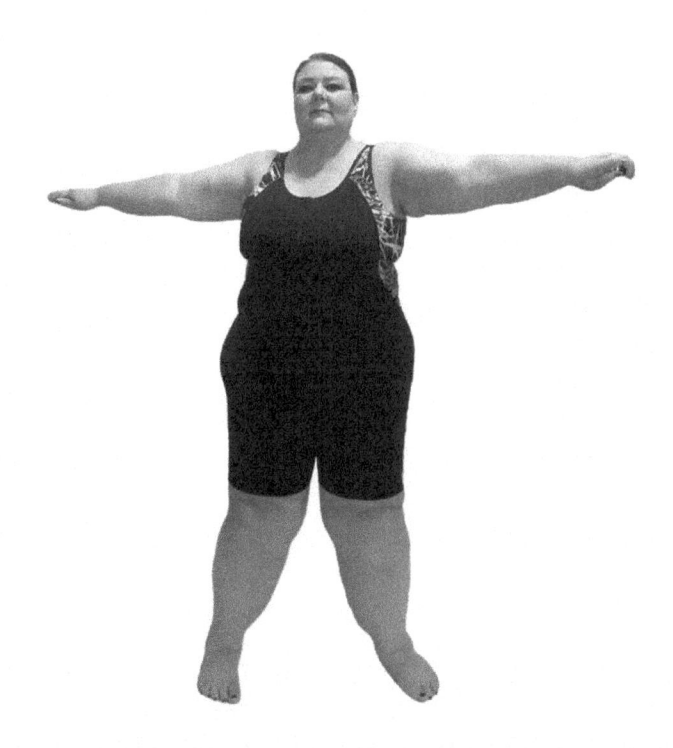

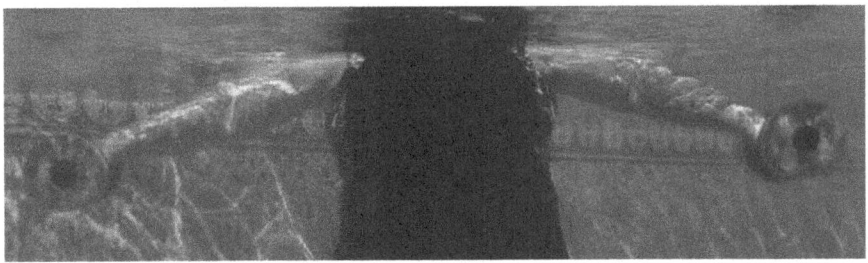

Deep water jumping Jacks.

Whole Body Exercises

Belly Dances: **Stand with your feet shoulder width apart. Make a circular motion with your hips and sway your hips from side to side and up and down while moving your arms in a hula like movement. So fun!**

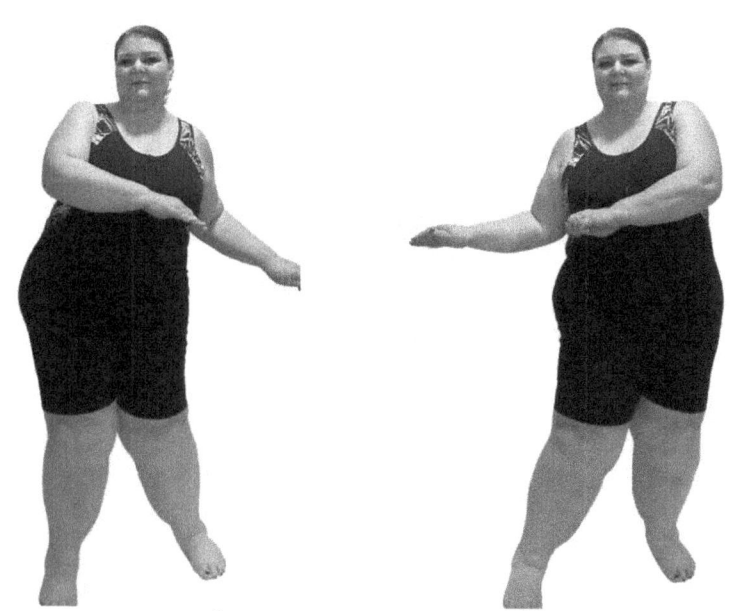

Belly Dance Starting and Mid Positions.

Hip Sways and Hip Rolls: **Basically, a belly dance but without the arms. Put your arms on your hips and pretend like you're that fun dancer on TV. No one's watching so have fun. It's great for your joints!**

Sassy Walk: **Sway your hips while taking steps more in front of your whole body, like a model on a catwalk would. Go for the big sway. Put your hands on your hips or swing your arms. Work it!**

Arm Exercises

Arm Circles, Forward and Backward: Make big circles in the water with your arms. For more challenge, make slower motions & bigger circles.

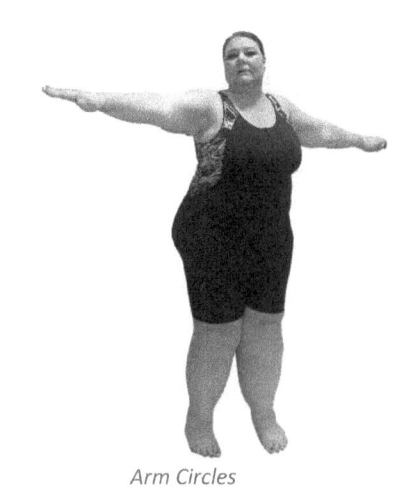

Arm Circles

Arm Claps Overhead – Better when done to fun music and big moves!

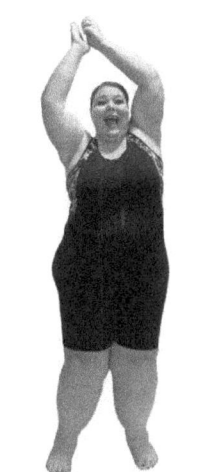

Arm Claps Overhead. Party on!

Arm Pulls – Gently hop forwards as you face both palms towards your chest and pull forward.

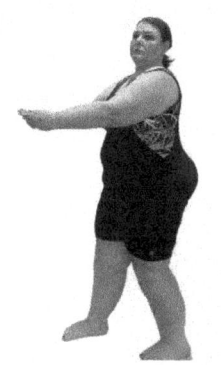

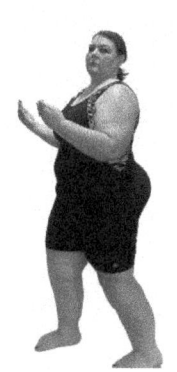

Arm Pulls starting and ending positions.

Arm Pushes: Gently hop backwards as you face your palms forward and push in front of you.

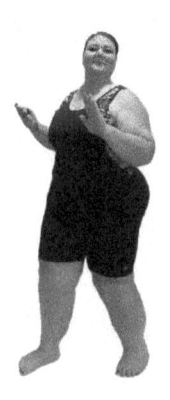

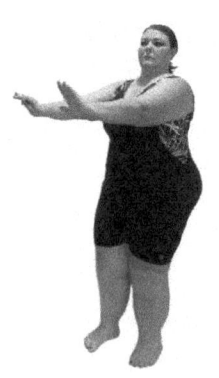

Pushes starting and ending positions.

Bicep Curls: I like to do these with aquatic dumbbells, but this would also be effective with a cupped hand or webbed glove.

1. Begin by standing straight with your feet shoulder-width apart, holding the water dumbbell in your right hand, ensuring that your palm is facing forward.
2. Position your arm close to your body, keeping your elbow stationary.
3. Slowly lift the dumbbell towards your shoulder, ensuring that only your forearm moves, while your upper arm remains stationary.
4. Hold the dumbbell at shoulder level for a moment, engaging your bicep muscle.
5. Carefully lower the dumbbell back to the starting position, ensuring that you maintain control throughout the movement.
6. Repeat this process for the desired number of repetitions, then switch to the left hand and repeat.
7. To maximize the effectiveness of the bicep curl, focus on maintaining good form and engaging your bicep muscle throughout the exercise.

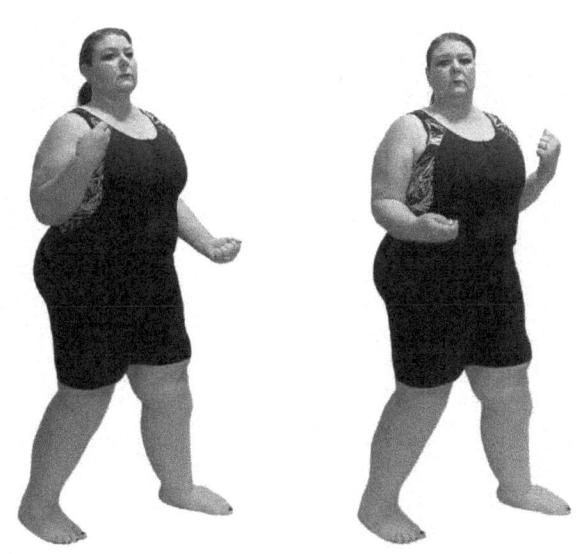

Bicep Curls starting and ending positions.

Chest:

1. Start by standing in waist-deep water.
2. Hold onto a foam noodle or pool dumbbells to create resistance.
3. Position your feet hip-width apart and engage your core muscles to maintain balance.
4. Bend your elbows and hold your arms to the sides.
5. Slowly bring your arms back towards your chest, keeping your palms facing together.
6. Push your arms out again until they are back beside the ears.

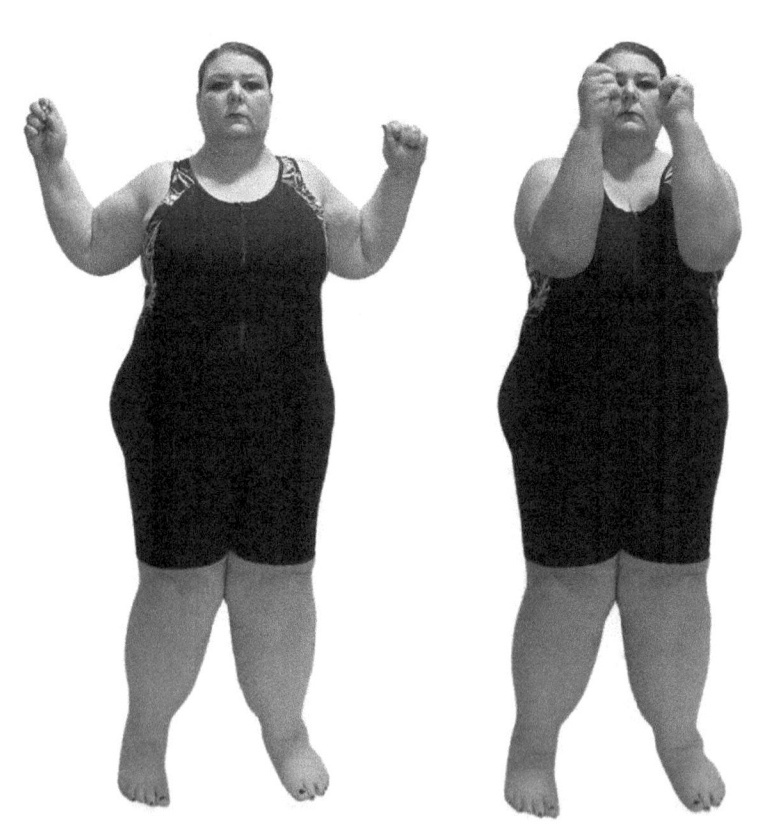

Chest exercises starting and ending positions. I normally perform this exercise with aquatic dumbbells at shoulder height water for maximum resistance.

Chest Turbulence: Like abdominal turbulence made by swooshing water up, you're just doing it higher and swooshing water down.

1. Stand in shallow water with your feet hip-width apart.
2. Place both hands in front of your chest, palms facing down.
3. Inhale deeply through your nose.
4. As you exhale forcefully through your mouth, push your hands down into the water as if you're trying to create ripples.
5. Continue this pattern of inhaling and exhaling while pushing your hands down to create turbulence in the water.

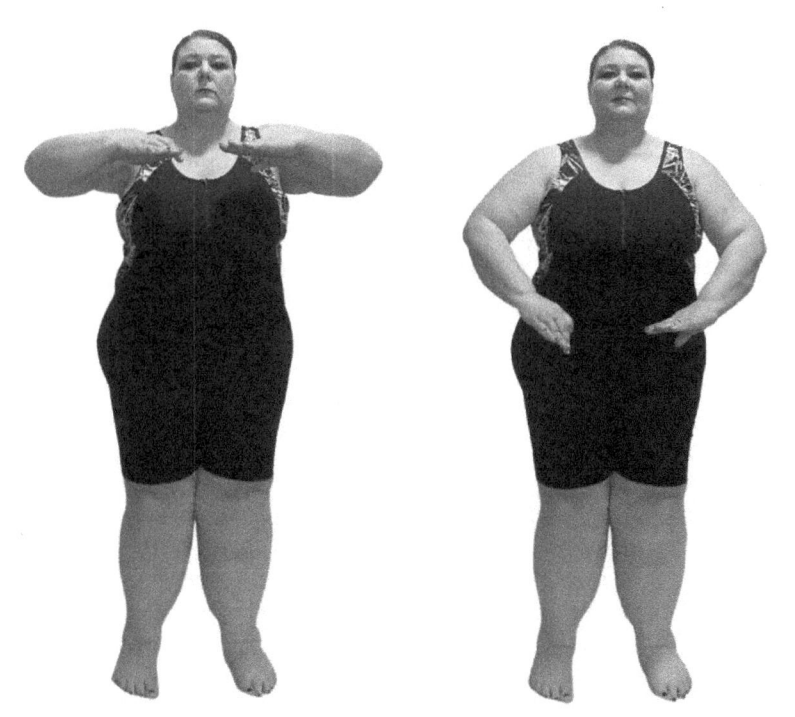

Swooshing water on your body to create Chest Turbulence, starting and mid positions.

Forward and Backwards Arm Rolls **Put both arms in front of you and roll them forwards for thirty seconds and then reverse direction for thirty seconds.** Great for lubricating the joints!

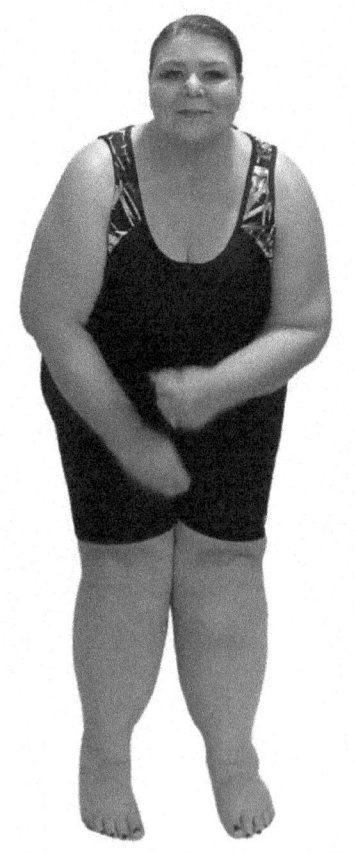

Forward and Backwards Arm Rolls

Punches

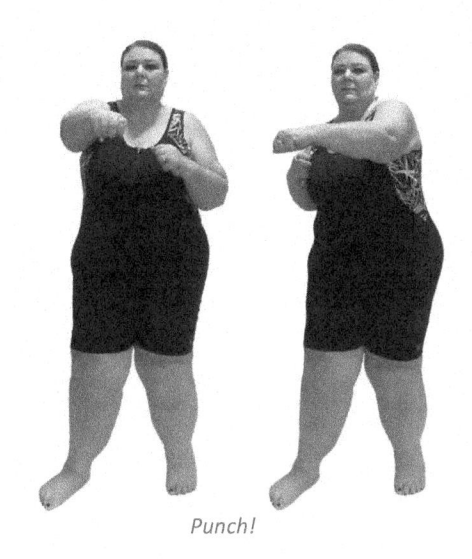

Punch!

Shoulder Rolls, Forward and Backwards: **Relax and roll shoulders up, back, down and forward letting your arms follow.**

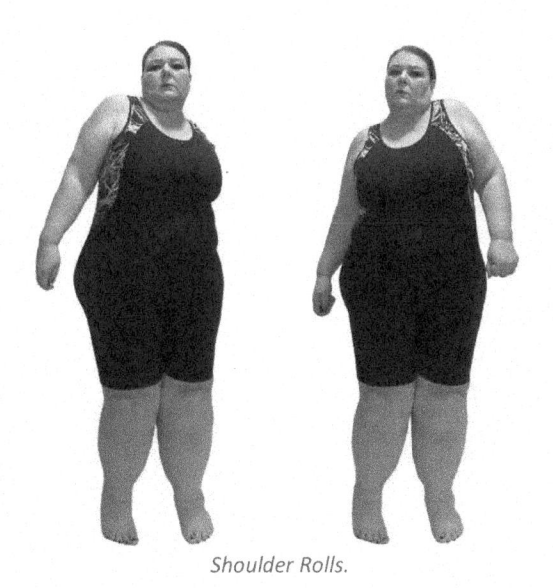

Shoulder Rolls.

Side Arm Lifts: I do these with aquatic dumbbells, but they would also be effective when you use your hands as resistance by cupping them. Starting with hands at your side, slowly raise them to the chest height and return to the side. Repeat 10-15 times.

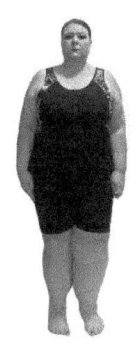

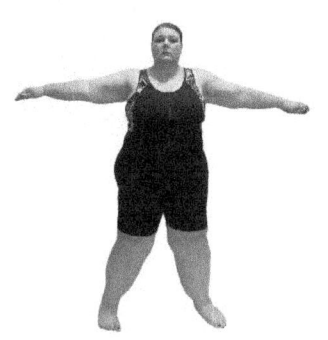

Side Arm Lifts starting and ending position.

Walking Breaststroke: **While walking, keep both hands pointed forward, and pushing them out to the side, walking forward in chest deep water.**

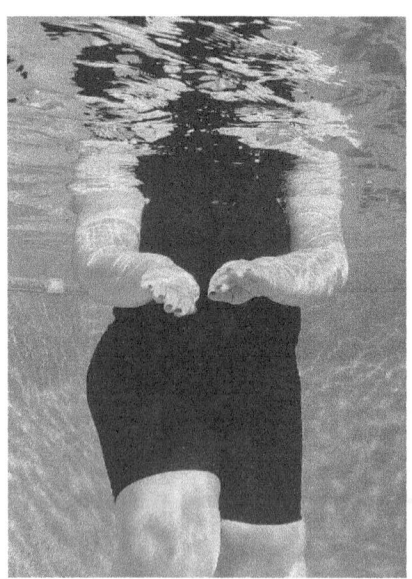

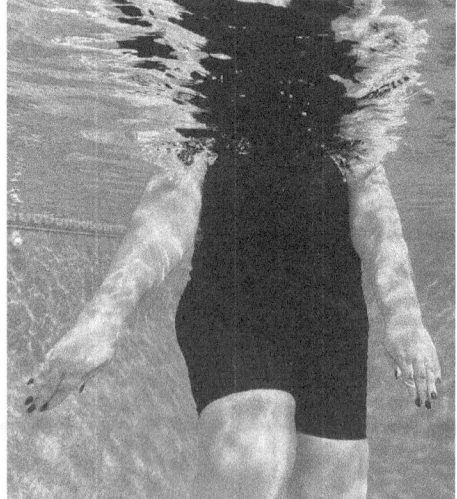

Walking Breaststroke.

Wall Pull Ups: You can do this when not touching or with your feet on the ground, moving up into a tippy toe. Grab on to the side with your palms facing the edge, and give a gentle pull, barely lifting out of the water.

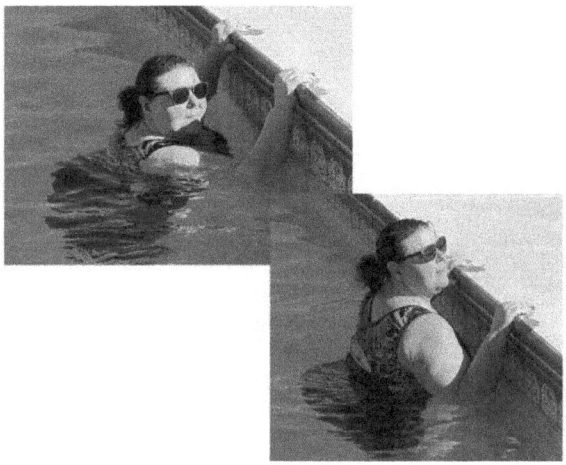

Wall Pull Ups.

Wall Push Ups: With your feet on the bottom of the pool. Spread your arms shoulder width apart and press your body towards the edge of the pool, gently, and push back out with your arms.

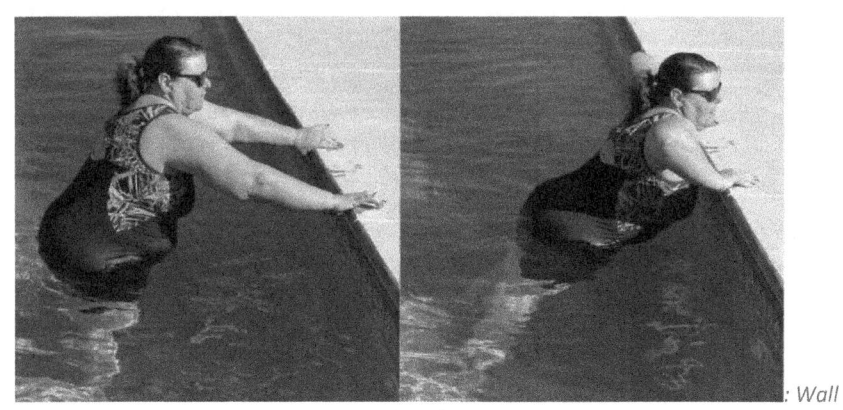

: Wall

Wall Push Ups.

Leg Exercises

Bicycles: **Alone, with a pool noodle or belt for flotation, or even dumbbells under the arms. Do them to the front, the right, and the left. You can even hang on to the side of the pool if you want. Just pedal away and ride that bicycle!**

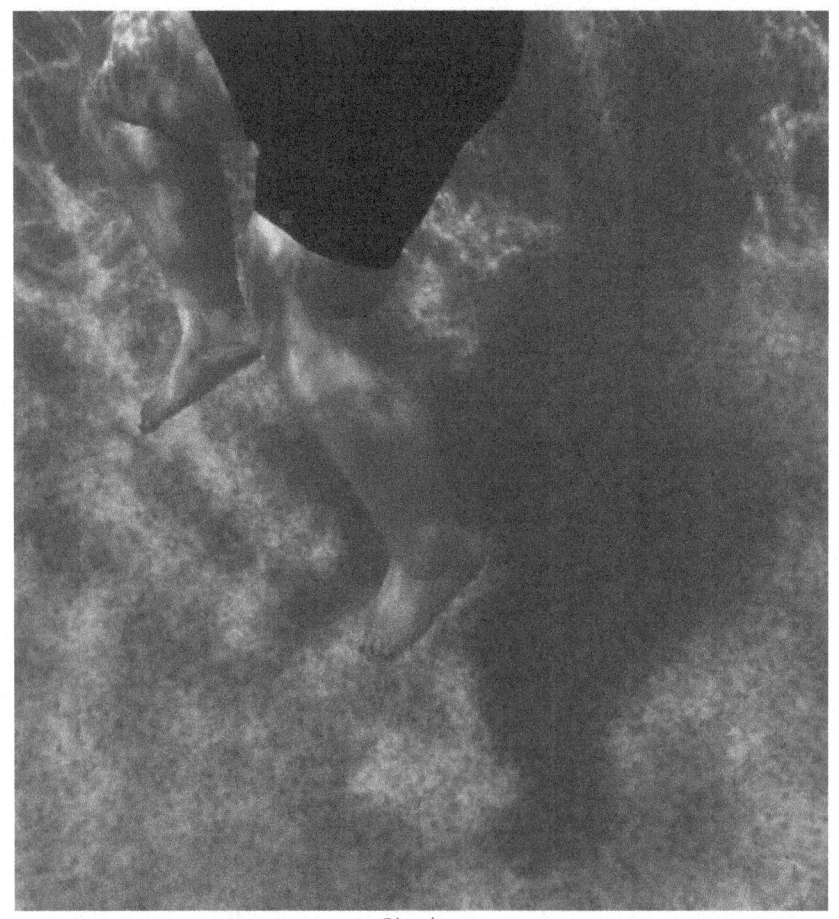

Bicycles.

Calf Raises on the Wall:

1. Stand with your feet hip-width apart and place your hands on a stable surface like a wall, chair back, or railing for support.
2. Slowly raise your heels off the ground, lifting your body weight onto the balls of your feet.
3. Keep your core engaged and your knees straight and hold the position for a few seconds at the top.
4. Lower your heels back down to the ground slowly.
5. Repeat for several repetitions as desired.

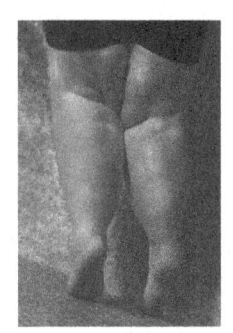

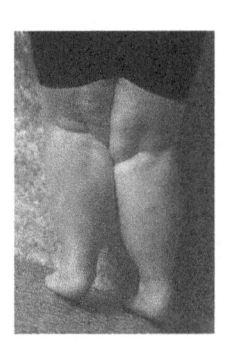

Calf Raises on the Wall starting and ending positions.

Circles of Feet: This exercise helps improve ankle flexibility and mobility.

1. Lift one foot and extend it in front of you.
2. Slowly rotate your foot clockwise in a circular motion.
3. Make sure to move your entire foot, including your toes and heel.
4. Repeat the circular motion 10-15 times.
5. Now rotate your foot counterclockwise for 10-15 repetitions.

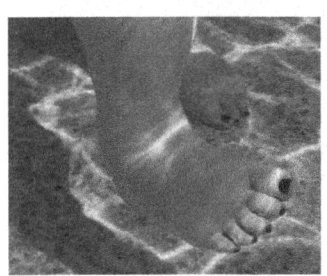

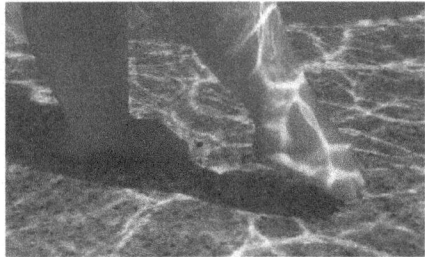

Circles of Feet.

Cross Country Skiing:

1. Begin by standing in waist-deep, or deeper water with your arms at your sides.
2. Lean forward slightly and lift your right knee toward your chest, keeping your foot flexed.
3. As you lift your right knee, extend your left leg backward, keeping it straight and parallel to the bottom of the pool.
4. Repeat this motion with your left leg, lifting it toward your chest as you extend your right leg backward.
5. Continue alternating legs in a fluid motion, mimicking the movement of cross-country skiing.
6. Focus on maintaining good form, keeping your core engaged, and breathing deeply as you move.
7. Gradually increase the speed and intensity of your movements to raise your heart rate and challenge your muscles.
8. Consider using resistance equipment such as water dumbbells or ankle weights to make the exercise more challenging.

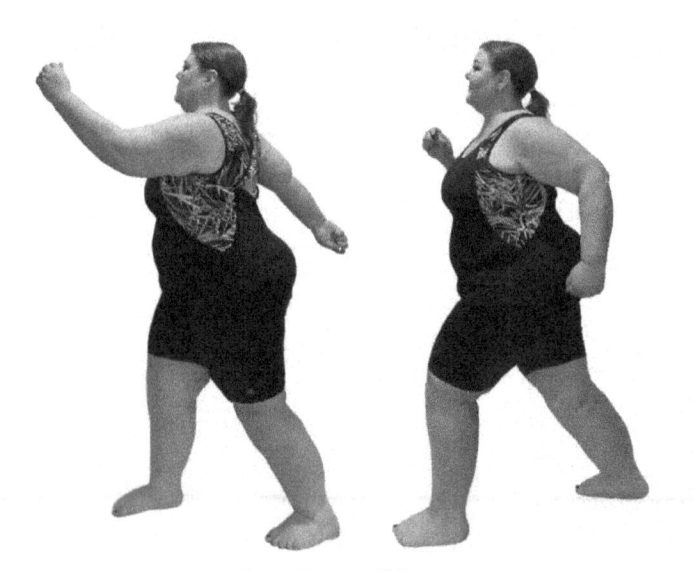

Cross Country Skiing.

Flutter Kicks using a Kickboard, Wall, or Dumbbells for Flotation:

1. Hold the kickboard out in front of you with both hands. If you're using dumbbells, place each bell under your armpits, and if you're using a wall, just hang onto the wall with your palms facing out and about shoulder width apart.
2. Keep your arms in front of you while holding the board and let your legs dangle down behind you.
3. Start kicking your legs up and down in a quick, alternating motion.
4. Keep your toes pointed and the movement should come from your hips, not your knees.
5. Maintain a steady, consistent rhythm with your kick.
6. Try to keep your body as straight as possible and avoid bending your knees too much.
7. Practice for a few minutes at a time and gradually increase the duration and intensity of your flutter kick.

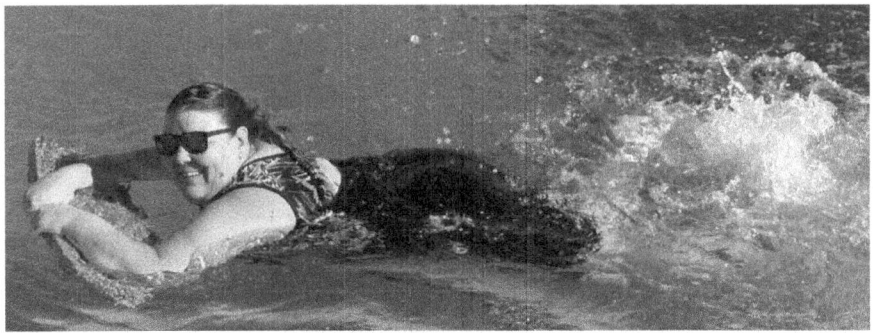

Flutter Kicks.

Forward to Backwards Kicks: **Holding onto a wall, kick one leg at a time forward, then back behind you, repeat ten times on each side.**

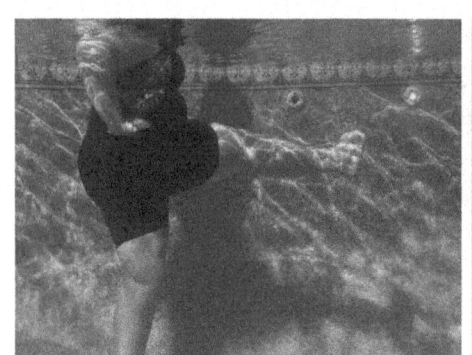

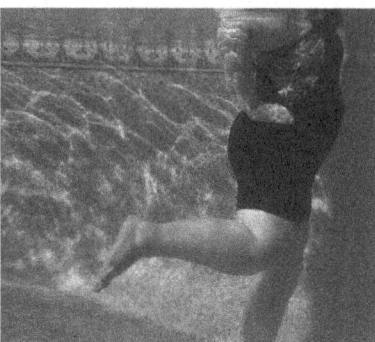

Forward to Backwards Kicks.

Forward Kicks (Can Cans): **You can do these either hanging onto a wall or freestyle. Make sure knee is straight and back stays straight. Don't bend to make the kick higher. Keep one foot planted while you kick forward, then alternate to the other leg. Repeat ten times.**

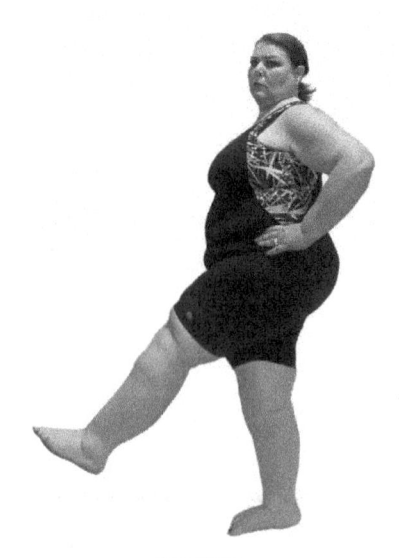

Can Cans.

Hip Hinge: Perform this in waist deep water, so you can breathe properly. This exercise is bending at the hips while keeping your spine straight and pushing your hips back. This improves posture, stability, and power in the lower body.

1. Stand with your feet shoulder-width apart, with your toes pointing forward.
2. Place your hands on your hips and keep your shoulders down and back. Next, engage your core muscles to stabilize your spine.
3. As you inhale, push your hips back and bend forward at the waist, keeping your back straight as you move. Focus on driving your hips backward, as opposed to bending your knees or rounding your spine.
4. Once you have reached your maximum range of motion, exhale and push through your heels to return to the starting position. Repeat the movement five times.

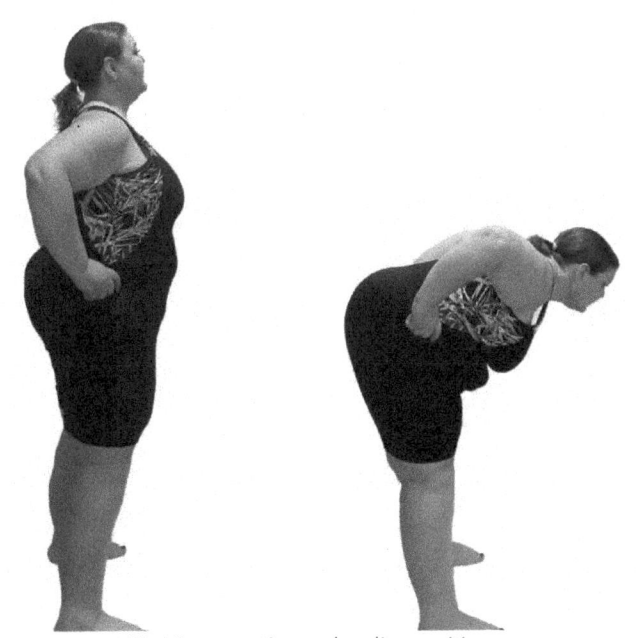

Hip Hinge starting and ending positions.

Knees to Chest: **Slow, fast, or riding on a pool noodle, think of this as water marching 101:** Alternate moving your knees to your chest (or as high as you can go), focusing on not overextending your hips.

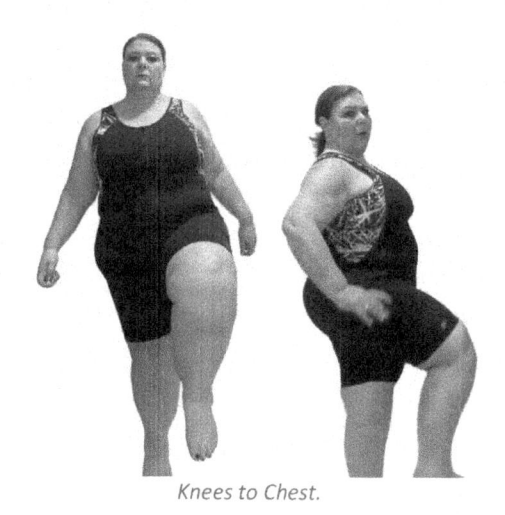

Knees to Chest.

Leg Extensions on Back, front, side:

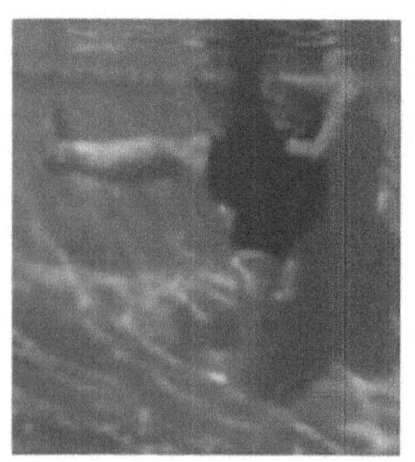

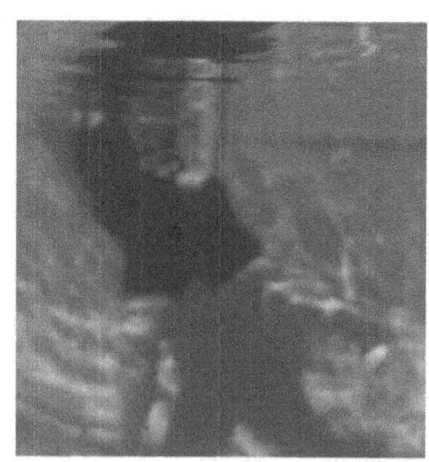

Leg Extensions.

Aqua Therapy for Lipedema and Lymphedema

Moguls:

1. Walk with your arms to the side, big like you're the boss!
2. As you walk, gently slap the front of the thigh. This touches on an area of lymph nodes and gives you the opportunity to move your arms big and bold!

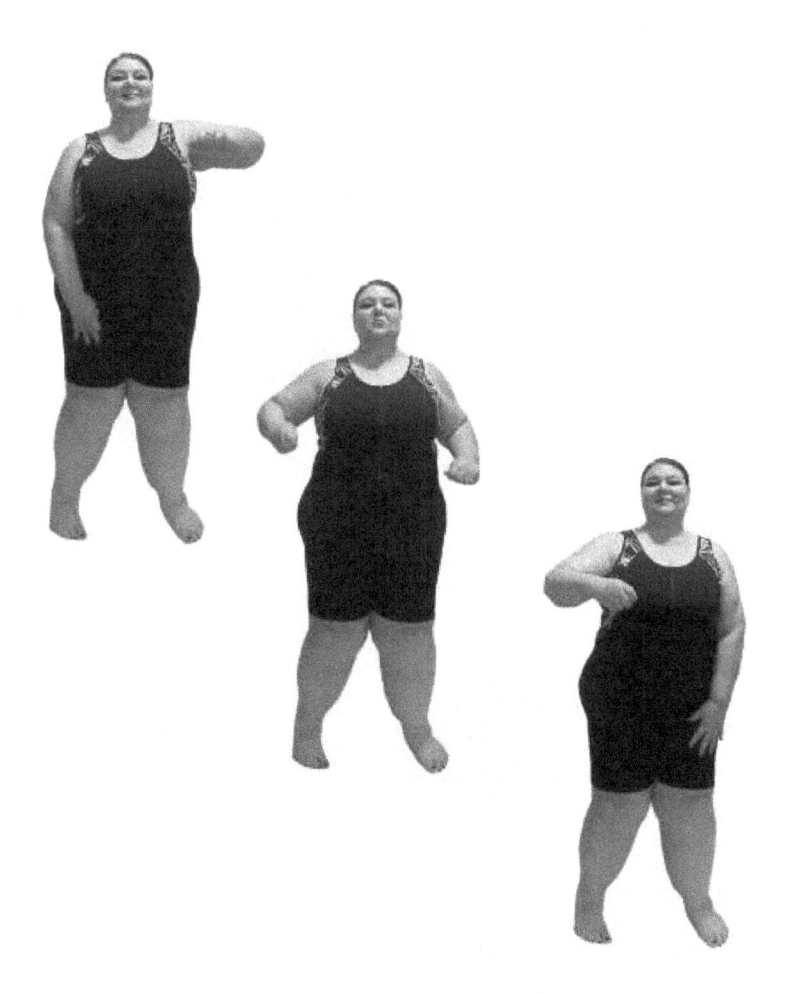

Moguls. Large and in charge!

Opening the Gate: **Lateral movements help with your hip flexibility and mobility. Perform in any depth of water, focusing on a soft landing.**

1. Stand with feet shoulder width apart.
2. Lift your right foot and move it to the side, as if opening a gate.
3. Bring your right foot back to the starting position.
4. Repeat with your left leg, opening the gate to the left side.
5. Continue alternating between your right and left foot.

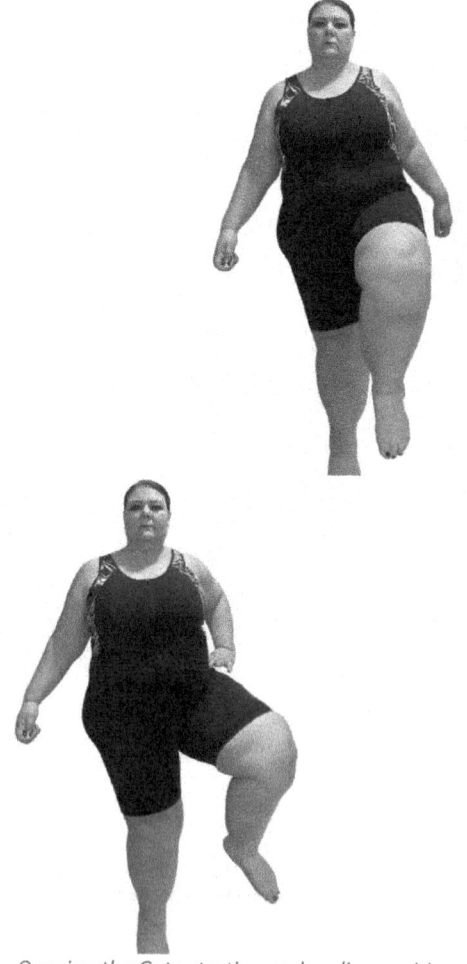

Opening the Gate starting and ending positions.

Aqua Therapy for Lipedema and Lymphedema

Out-out, In-ins (Tire Running Exercise): **OK I made that name up.** Pretend you're in football player training camp, with a line of tires in front of you to run in. I like to do this when I'm floating freely.

1. Put one foot directly in front of you (like it's going inside the tire)
2. Now put the other foot IN the tire.
3. Now step out of your imaginary tire with a big step to the outside.
4. Step the other foot out of the 'tire' with a big step to the outside.
5. So, your feet are going out, out, in in, out, out, in in repeatedly.
6. This can be done in waist deep water too, but I think it's harder in the shallow end.

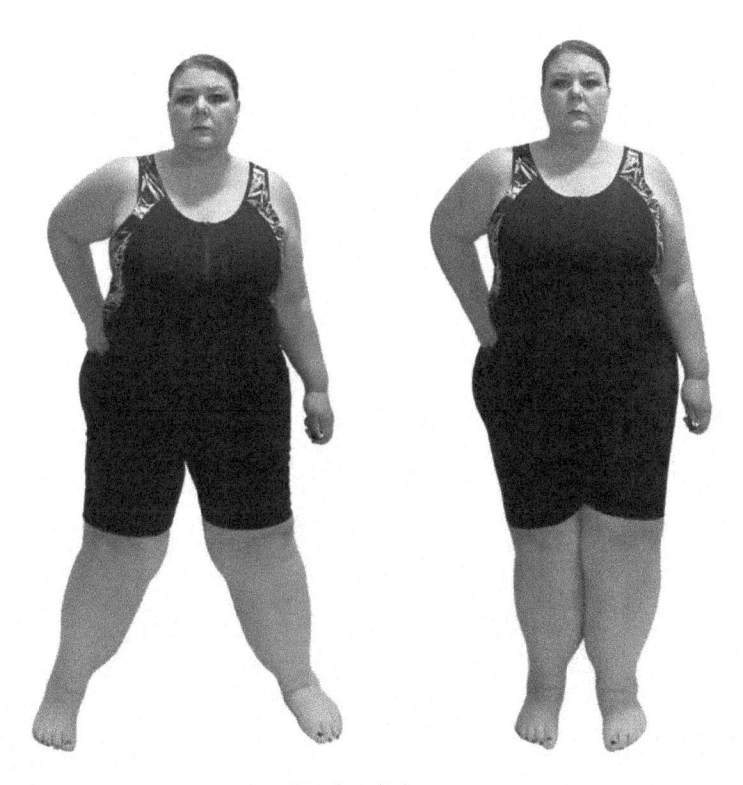

Out-Out, In-Ins.

Pool Noodle Car Clutches: **This is pretending that your foot is pushing the clutch of a car, but on top of a pool noodle. It's tricky, but a good leg strengthening exercise.**

1. Twist, finagle, and wiggle until your foot is on the middle of the pool noodle.
2. Hold each end of the pool noodle in your hands as you raise and lower your leg.
3. Switch legs and try to keep the pool noodle from popping out of the water by controlling your leg motion. Raise and lower your leg as you control the noodle.
4. After a few car clutches, switch legs and repeat. It's fun!

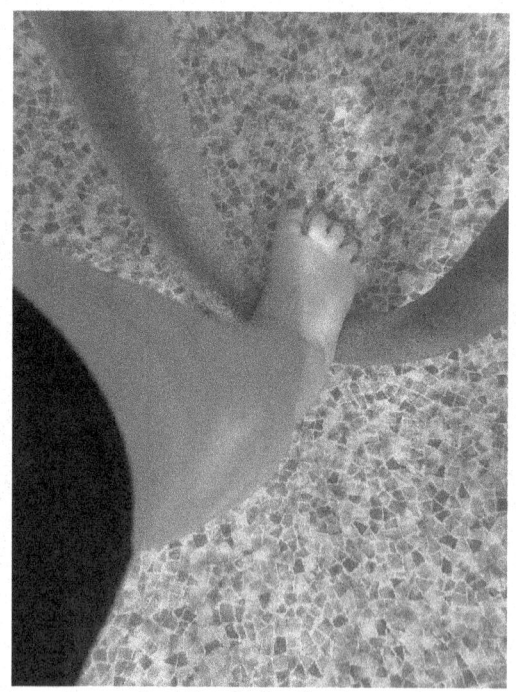

Pool Noodle Car Clutches.

Scissor Kicks: I believe this exercise really moves my lymph. I try to speed up as I'm doing them. This is the same leg motion as for cross country, but to the sides.

1. Stand in chest-deep or deeper water, keeping your back straight and tummy as tight as you can. Hold on to the edge if you like!
2. Put your arms out to the side for balance, if you need to.
3. Start by keeping legs straight and together. But point your toes!
4. Open your legs to the sides, and cross them over each other, alternating which leg is on top with repetitions, like scissors.
5. You can do small or big motions on this one. I like to really get in the deep end and do giant scissor kicks, both horizontally and vertically.
6. Keep your head and chest up throughout the exercise.

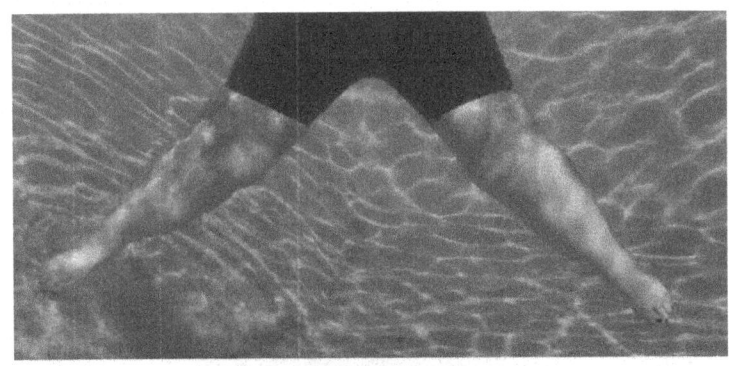

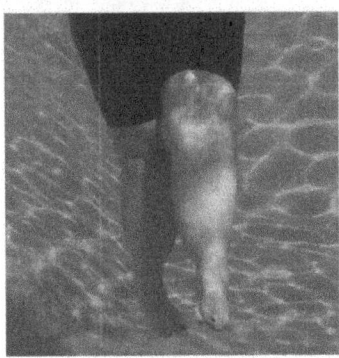

Scissor Kicks.

Toe Clenches: Curl your toes and squeeze them for about three seconds, then relax toes for three seconds. Repeat three times on each foot.

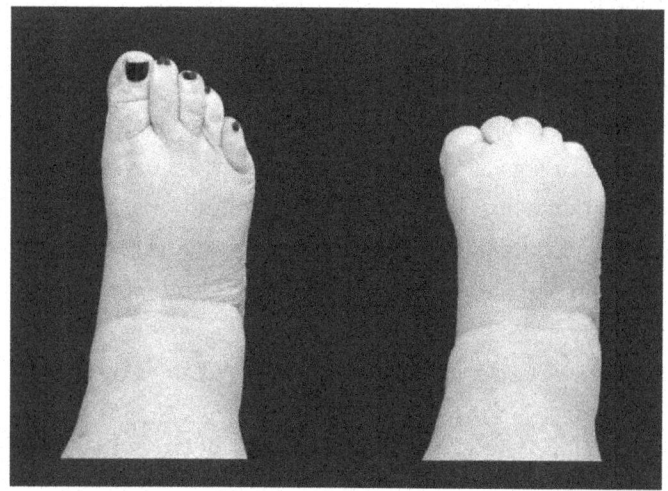

Toe Clenches.

Toe Spreads): Spread your toes as far as possible and hold for three seconds, then relax toes for three seconds.

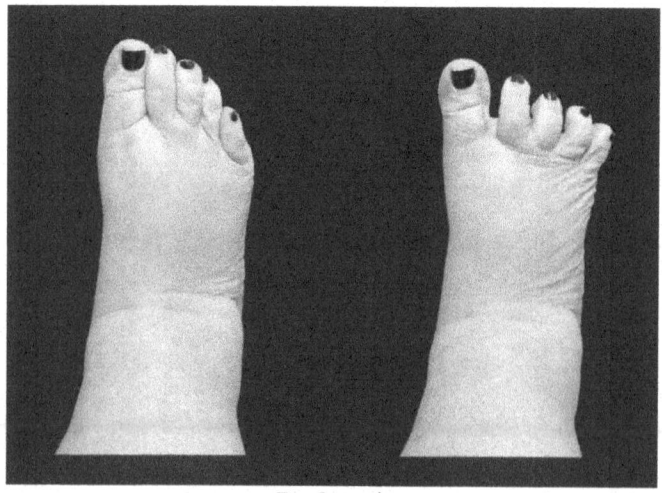

Toe Spread.

Walking on your Tippy Toes: This can be done in up to chest deep water.

1. Stand up with feet shoulder width apart.
2. Raise your heels off the ground, lifting your body onto the balls of your feet.
3. Balance on your tippy toes, keep your tummy tight if you can.
4. Take fifteen steps forward and try to keep your balance.
5. Remember to keep your head and chest up on this one, and shoulders back. Don't lean forward.

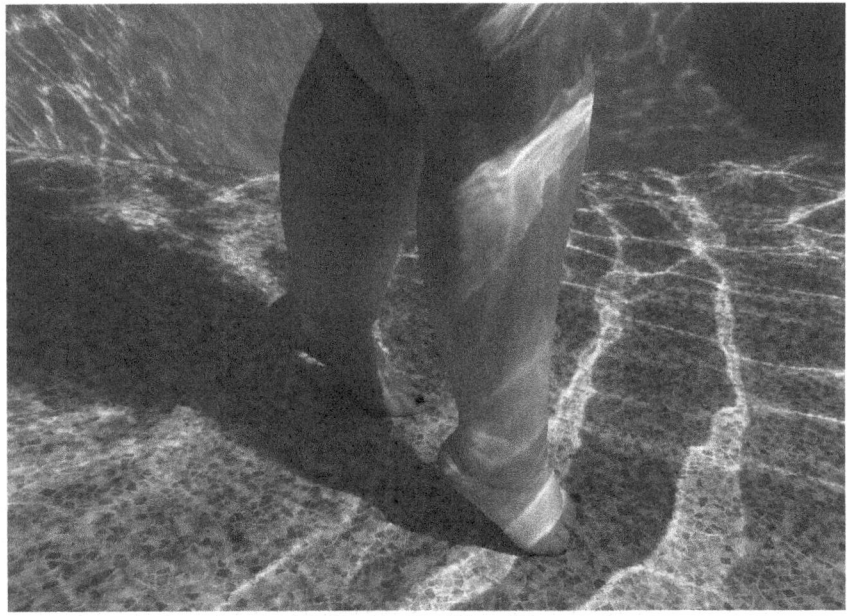

Walking on Your Tippy Toes.

Wall Touches: Done while holding onto the side of the pool.

1. With one side of your body against the pool, extend the leg farthest from the wall in front of you, and swing it gently to the pool wall and touch.
2. Now swing that leg all the way behind you and touch the wall with your toe behind you. It may take months of this movement to be able to touch the wall. Progress, not perfection!
3. Do this six times, then repeat with the other leg.

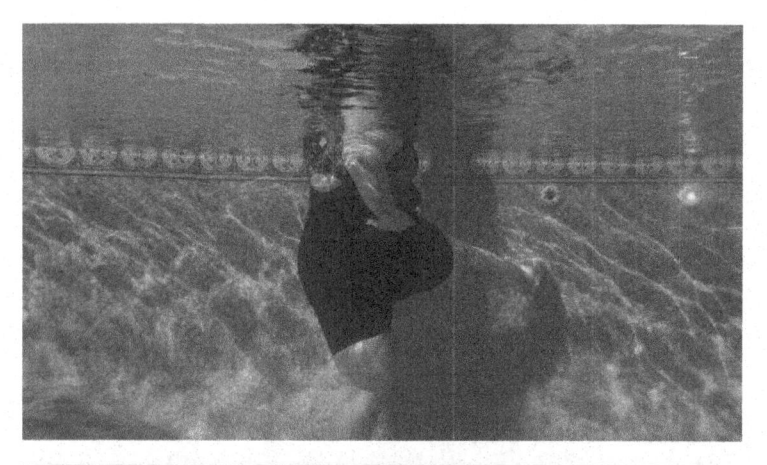

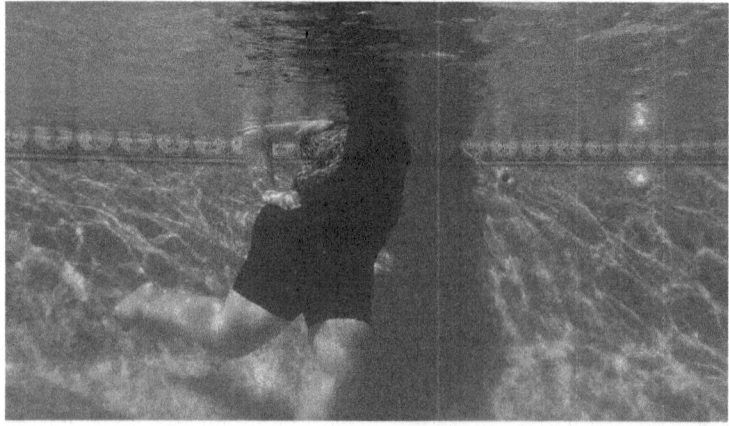

Wall Touches Starting and Mid Positions.

Stretching Exercises

I prefer to do my stretching at the end of a session as a part of a cool down and relax time, and I water walk for my warmup. Stretching is important to help with flexibility and reduce soreness. Here are a few I really like. Note that I do all stretching in chest deep or shallower water, where I can touch the bottom of the pool.

Arm Sways: So relaxing! This is one of my favorite cooldown stretches done in a slow, flowing motion.

1. Stand in chest-deep water with your feet shoulder-width apart and your arms at your sides.
2. Take a deep breath in, and as you exhale, raise both arms out to the sides, keeping them straight and parallel to the surface of the water.
3. Inhale and as you exhale, slowly bring your arms forward, crossing them in front of your body at chest level.
4. Continue to exhale as you slowly move your arms out to the sides again, keeping them straight and parallel to the surface of the water.
5. Repeat the arm sway stretch 5-10 times, moving slowly and smoothly through each repetition.

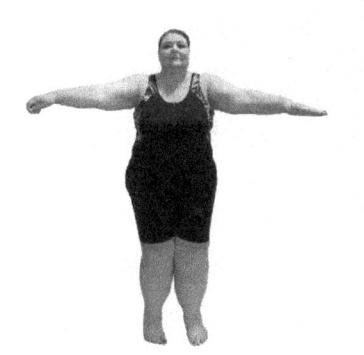

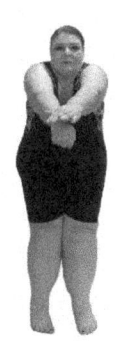

Arm Sways.

Arm Overhead Stretch (Triceps Stretch): **A simple stretch to relieve shoulder, neck, and upper back tension.**

1. Stand up straight with your feet shoulder-width apart.
2. Raise your left arm straight up overhead, reaching towards the sky with your fingertips.
3. With your right hand, grasp your left elbow and gently pull it towards your right side, feeling the stretch in your left shoulder and upper back.
4. Hold the stretch for 15-30 seconds, breathing deeply and relaxing into the stretch.
5. Release the stretch and repeat on the other side, raising your right arm overhead and grasping your right elbow with your left hand.

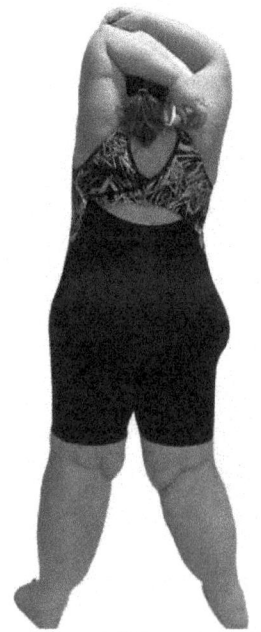

Arm Overhead Stretch (Triceps Stretch).

Bicep Stretch:

1. Stand with your feet shoulder-width apart and reach one arm straight out in front of you with your palm facing up.
2. Use your other hand to gently pull your fingers back towards your wrist, feeling the stretch in your bicep. Hold the stretch for 15-30 seconds, then release.
3. Repeat on the other side.

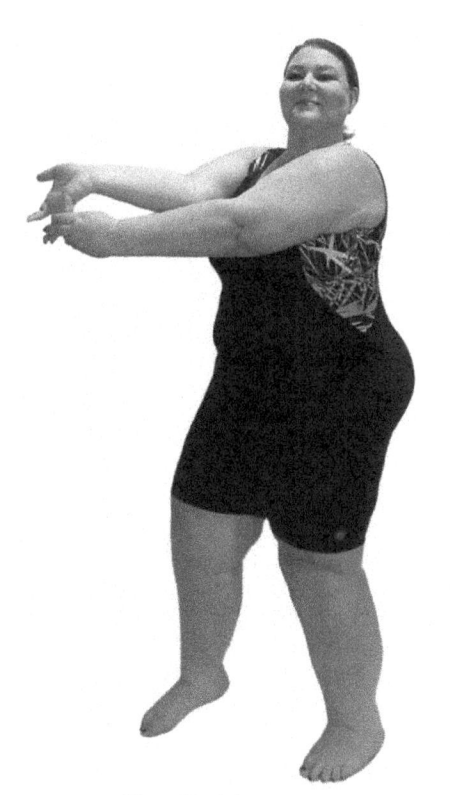

Bicep Stretch.

Big Self Hug: **No explanation needed!**

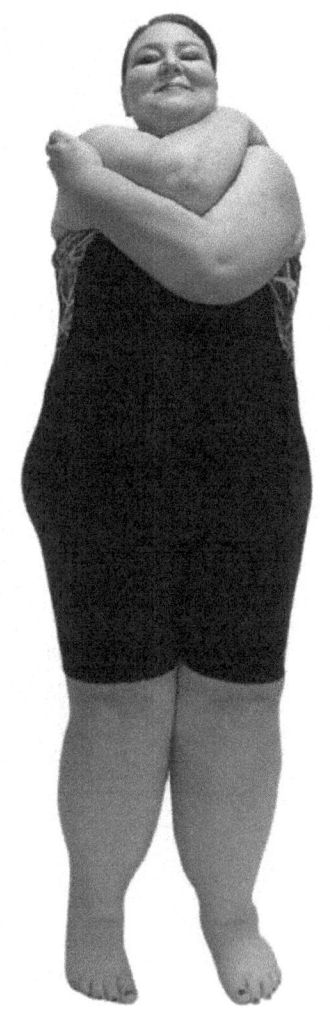

A Big Self Hug – You Deserve it!

Chest Stretch:

1. Stand with your feet shoulder-width apart and clasp your hands together in front of your chest.
2. Slowly push your hands away from your body, feeling the stretch in your chest and shoulders.
3. Hold the stretch for 15-30 seconds, then release.

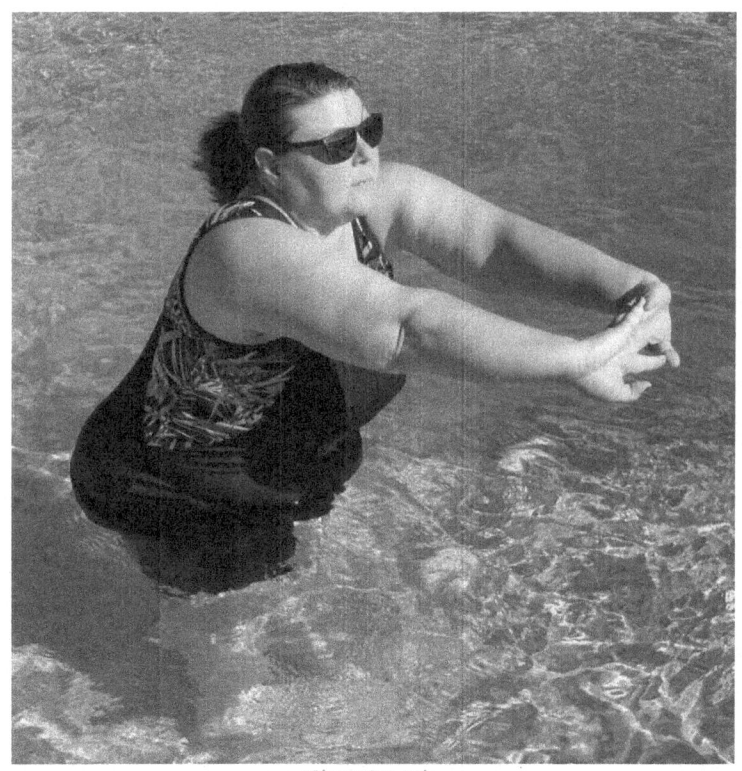

Chest Stretch.

Hamstring Stretch, Standing.

1. Stand in waist-deep water and hold onto the edge of the pool or use a pool noodle for support.
2. Extend one leg in front of you, placing heel on the ground. This is the leg you will be stretching.
3. Slowly lift your toe as high as you can while keeping the leg straight. You should feel a stretch in the back of your thigh.
4. To add a bit of oomph, raise both of your arms over your head.
5. Hold this position for 10-20 seconds, or longer if you can.
6. Repeat on the other side.

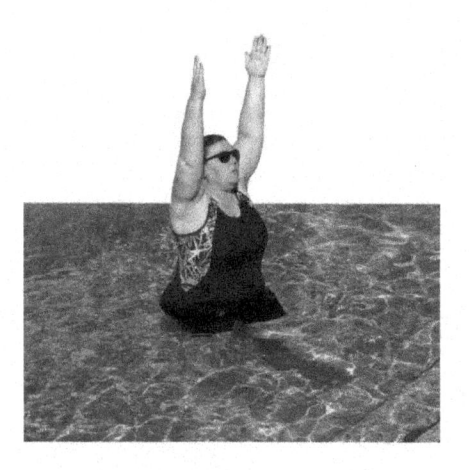

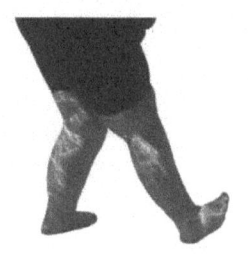

Hamstring Stretch, Standing.

Hamstring Stretch, Sitting

1. Sit on the steps or edge of the pool.
2. Extending your leg out in front of you, with your heels resting on the bottom of the pool or on a step.
3. Lean forward to feel a stretch in your hamstring.

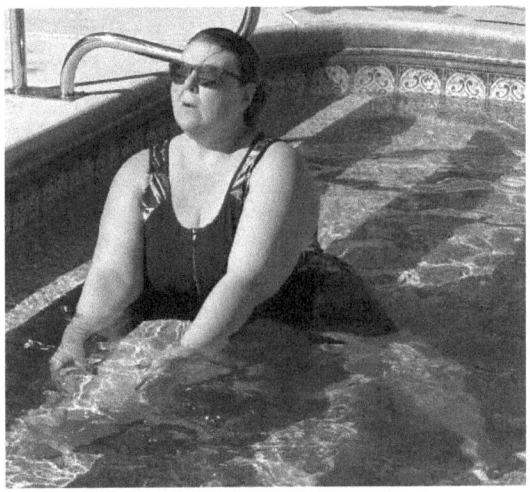

Hamstring Stretch, Sitting.

Head turns, side to side and stretch: **Turn left and right, and gently stretch.**

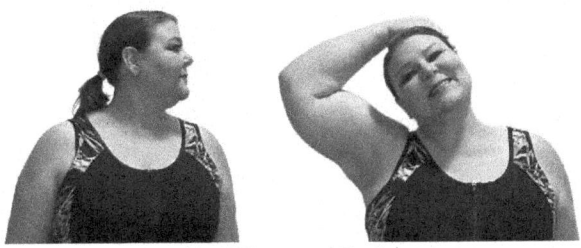

Head Turns and Stretches.

Push and Pull the Beach Ball (Or kickboard or floatie): **Done standing.** Put the ball right at the water line to get good resistance as you push and pull several times. .

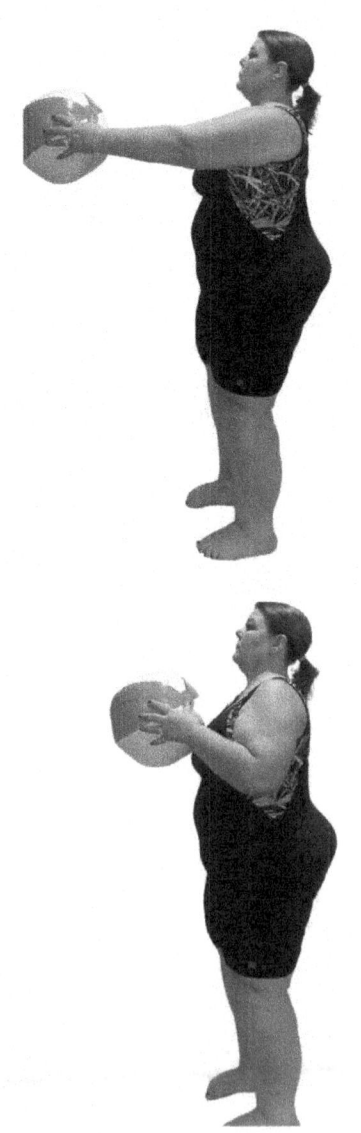

Push and Pull the Beach Ball.

Reaching to the Sky

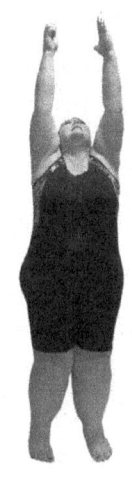

Reach to the Sky!

Shoulder Raises: **A little shoulder lift, scrunching the shoulder toward the ears, held for two counts, relax for 2 counts.**

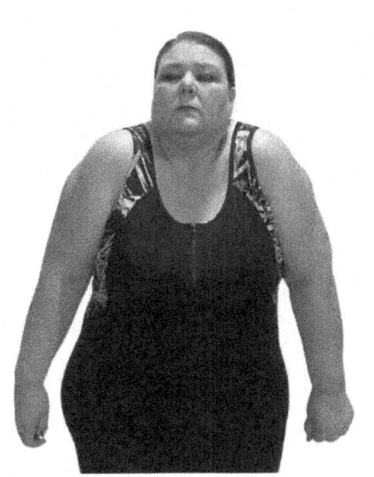

Shoulder Raises.

Side Arm Stretch: **Perform standing with non-stretched arm holding onto the pool edge** Hold each stretch for 15-30 seconds. Repeat on Both Sides.

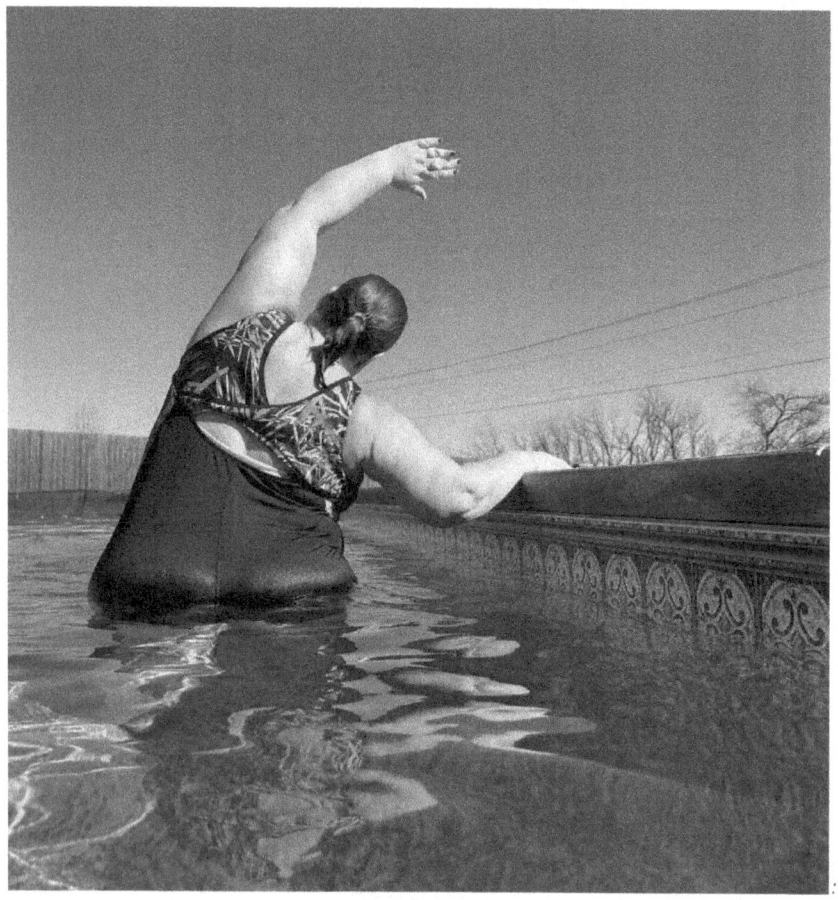

Side Arm Stretch.

Squats on the Wall (don't do this if it hurts your knees:

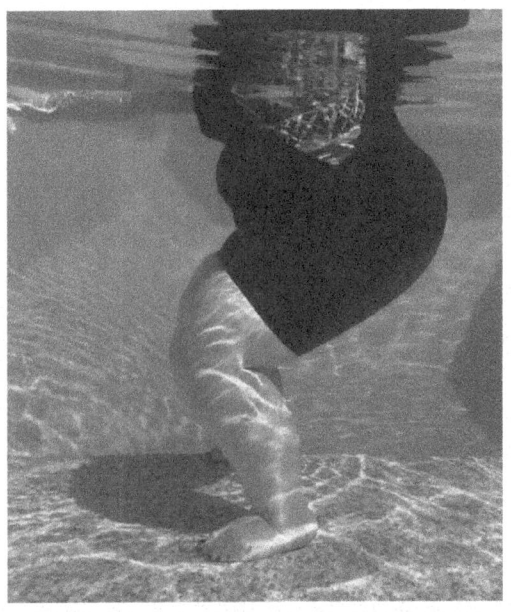

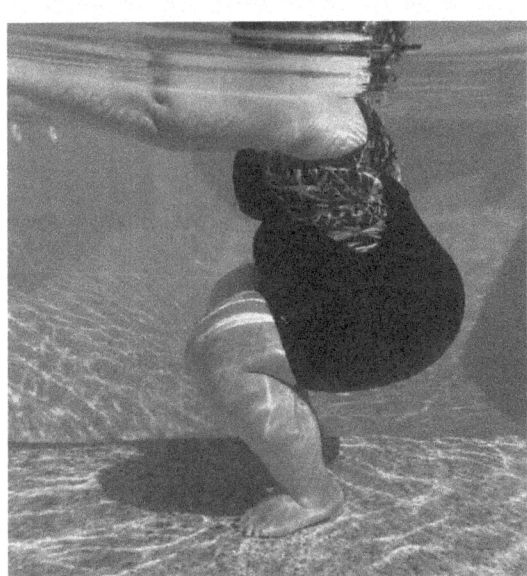

Squats on the Wall.

Standing Leg Circles on the Wall: **Perform these while standing on each leg, making big circles forwards and backwards. Repeat six times on each leg while holding onto the pool edge.**

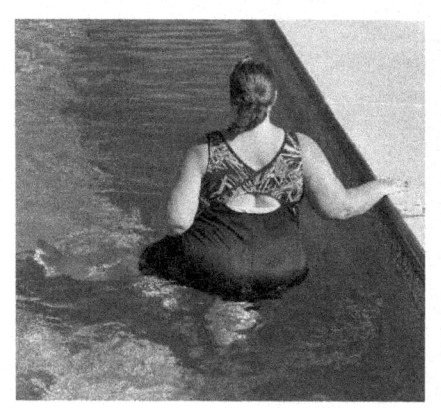

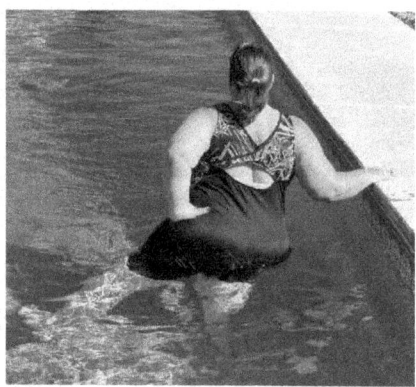

Standing Leg Circles.

Triceps Stretch: **(See Arm Overhead Stretch, p.138 for description).**

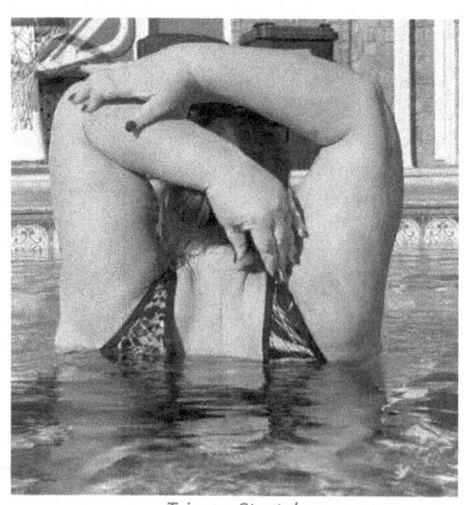

Triceps Stretch

Yoga Pose – Floating Savasana: **Float on your back with your arms and legs extended and do your abdominal breathing. Relax and unwind!!!**

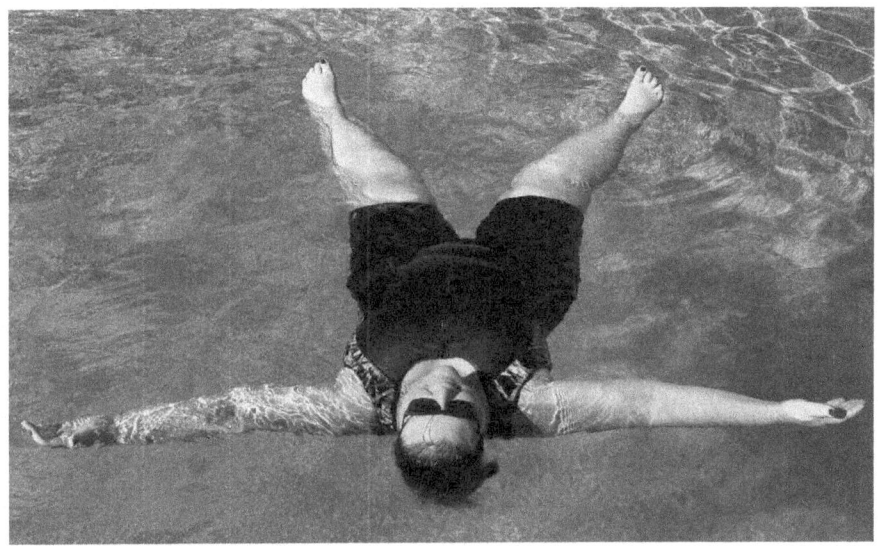

Floating Savasana

Yoga Pose – Water Chair:

1. Stand in waist-deep water and press your back against the side of the pool.
2. Lower your hips until your thighs are lower (try to get them parallel to the pool floor as you make progress), like you're sitting in a chair.
3. Hold the position for three deep breaths.
4. Slowly stand back up, or swim away!

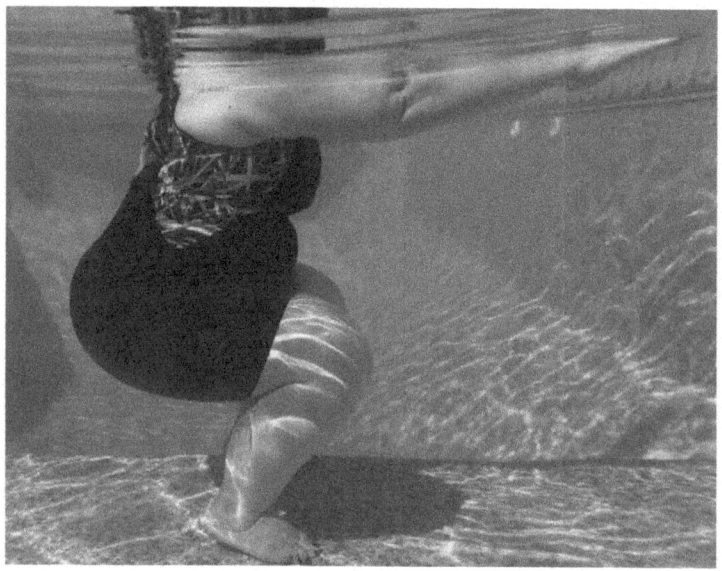

Water Chair Pose

Yoga Pose – Water Child's Pose: This only works in some pools. You'll have to try it to see if your pool edge is the right high (close to the waterline).

1. Stand in waist deep water, facing the pool's edge.
2. Sink down slowly until your arms and head rest on the edge of the pool. Try to feel a small stretch in your back.
3. Breathe deeply ad relax your body.

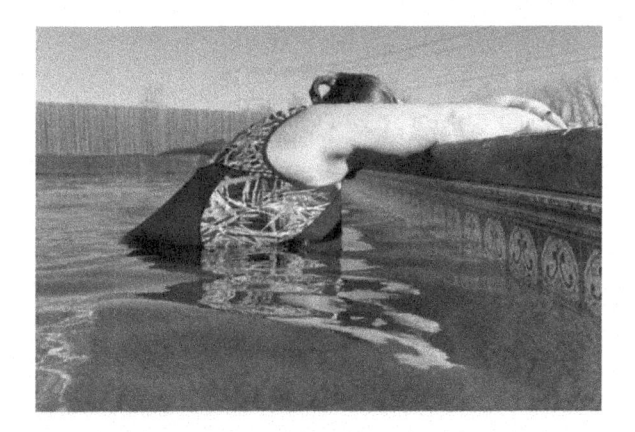

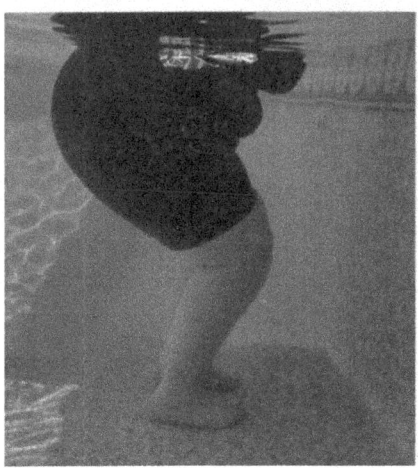

Water Child's Pose

Yoga Pose – Water Tree Pose: **Focus on a point outside the pool. This is a pose I cannot do on land, but in the water, it is glorious!**

1. From standing in waist-deep water, lift your right foot off the bottom of the pool.
2. Place the sole of the right foot against the inside of your left leg (some people can go as high as the thigh but go for what feels comfortable). Press firmly.
3. Bring your hands together in front of your heart and hold the pose.
4. Hold as long as you'd like.
5. Try versions of this pose while holding onto the pool edge if your balance is challenging at first.

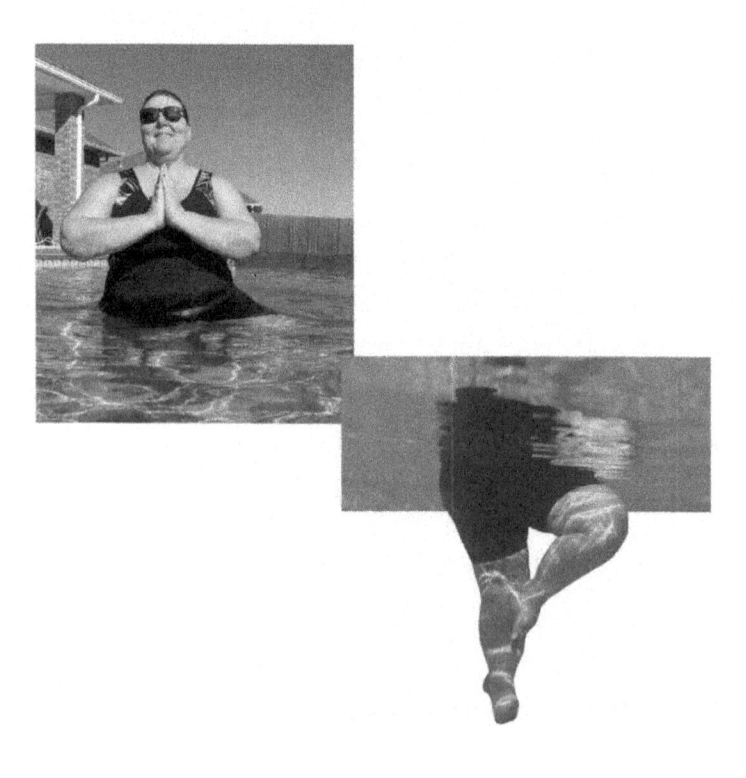

Water Tree Pose.

Pelvic Floor Exercises

Many women who have lipedema experience urinary stress incontinence. The correlation between lipedema and incontinence hasn't been solidified, but researchers are leading to some early conclusions that it is because of the connective tissues being compromised in the body. The health of the pelvic floor is important to everyone though. We need this part of the body to be strong to help us cough, sneeze, vomit, have sex, urinate, defecate, lift, walk and run and so on. And what feels most important to many of us is that it helps us be strong enough to not wet our pants involuntarily! .

Exercising your pelvic floor is important way to keep your hygiene and quality of life up! You may not have thought about it before, but performing your pelvic floor exercises in the water is a great idea. This is because of the effects of buoyancy that remove pressure from your lower body in the water. And with the extra resistance of water, you can get the job done with less repetitions and shorter session time of your pelvic floor exercises, and that makes the water a perfect environment to do this type of work.

IMPORTANT: Make sure your bladder is empty before you do pelvic floor exercises!

When you're doing your Kegels in the water, feel free to hang onto a pool noodle, the edge of the pool, or other floating device to aid you in support. And remember to keep your butt muscles (glutes) untightened while you Kegel away.

How to do Kegel Exercises

With an empty bladder, tighten your pelvic floor muscles and hold 3-5 seconds. Relax for 3-5 seconds and repeat 10 times. Do this every morning, afternoon, and night. If you can get one session in the water, that's a little bit easier Kegel time.

And for everyone's benefit, I will not be making an image to reference. You may have to Google this one if you need help learning Kegels. I know you understand!

Sample Workouts

Water Walking Routine

1. Deep breathing for a minute.
2. Walk in waist-high water for five minutes forwards. It's OK to hold onto a kickboard or dumbbells to keep your arms on the water if you want.
3. Walk in waist-high water for two minutes backwards.
4. Walk using a right-side step for one minute.
5. Walk using a left side step for one minute.
6. Walk forward using the biggest steps you can take for one minute.
7. Now, go a tiny bit faster and walk forwards for two more minutes.
8. Stop for deep abdominal breathing for one minute.
9. Abdominal massage one minute.
10. Very slow walk for two minutes.
11. Do very small ankle circles on each leg 5-7 times each way.
12. Do ten calf raises while holding onto the wall.
13. Stretch both arms to the sky, getting a good stretch in the arms, band torso.
14. One last big, deep breath as you bring arms to the sides.
15. Now float around and relax!

Aqua Jogging Routine

1. Deep breathing for a minute.
2. Massage legs for a minute.
3. Walk 5-7 minutes in any depth deeper than waist.
4. Jog for one to two songs, at whatever pace feels good (knees high, like I'm stepping over something).
5. Walk or tread water for a minute.
6. Massage legs and deep breathing for a minute.
7. Jog for another two to four songs, a little harder, but not so much that I'm feeling the burn.
8. Massage legs and deep breathing for a minute.
9. Walk 5-7 minutes.
10. Stand on one foot and flex ankles, then do ankle circles.

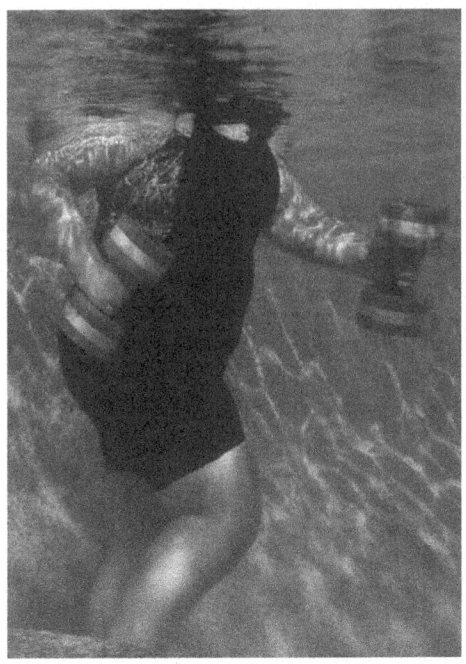

Aqua Jogging.

My Chill Day Routine

Some days, I just 'be' in the water for free and natural compression and some down time. I keep my legs below me (vertical) and not on the water for maximum compression.

Then again, some days at the end of a session, I float on my back and do deep breathing and talk to the stars.

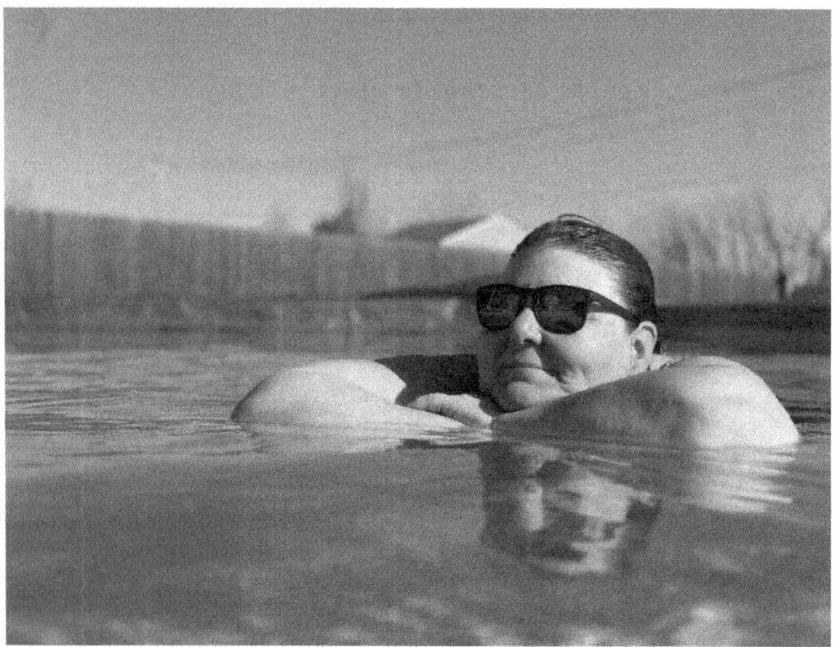

A Serious Chill Day Routine: Excellent for Stress and Swelling Reduction!

Deeper Water Routine

1. Deep breathing for a minute.
2. Abdominal massage for a minute.
3. Leg massage for a minute.
4. Walk for two minutes, slowly in at least waist high water.
5. Jog in place in deeper water now, for two minutes. Any speed.
6. Do ten scissor kicks.
7. Do ten cross country skis.
8. Bicycle for two minutes.
9. Deep breathing for a minute.
10. Abdominal massage for a minute.
11. Flutter kick for a minute.
12. Do ten scissor kicks.
13. Hold on to a wall, do ten forward/backward kicks on each leg.
14. Hold onto a wall, do six forward and six backwards circles on each leg.
15. Hold onto a wall, do ten wall touches in front of, then behind you.
16. Hold onto a wall, now in shallower water, do ten calf raises.
17. Walk two minutes.
18. Leg massage for two minutes.
19. End with deep abdominal breathing for a minute.

IMPORTANT: Remember to relax and enjoy your time in the water!

"They both listened silently to the water, which to them was not just water, but the voice of life, the voice of Being, the voice of perpetual Becoming."

~ Hermann Hesse ~

Resources and Support

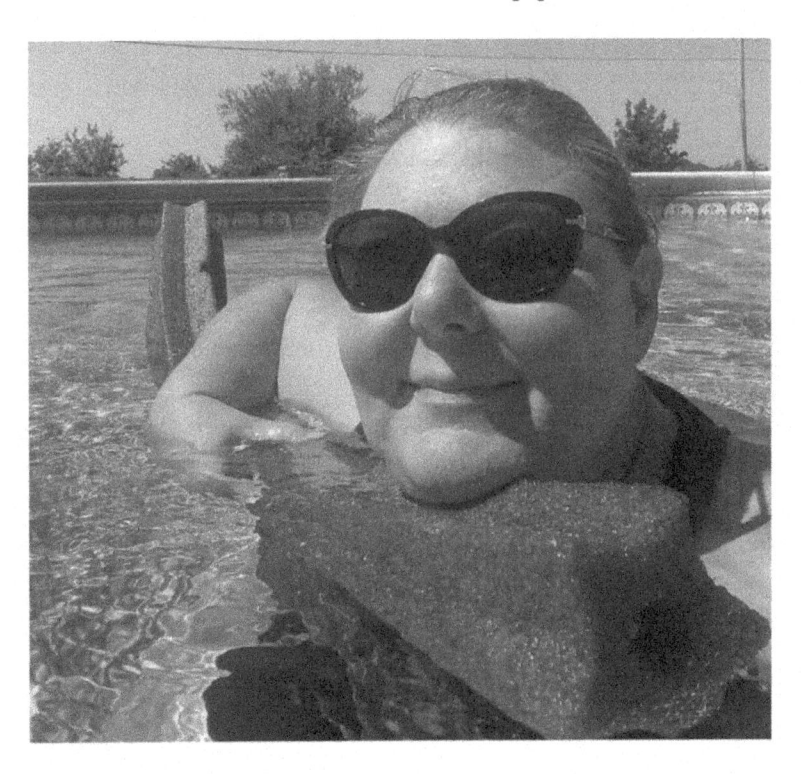

Chapter 10: Resources and Support

There are all kinds of organizations out there that support aquatic therapy. Here are just a few ideas for places you could go to get support:

- Aqua therapy and Rehab Institute / Aquatic Exercise Association AEA-CEC

QR Link to Aqua therapy and Rehab Institute

- LegsLikeMine.com
- Facebook Groups:
- Lipedema Lymphedema Water Exercise Mermaids
- Your local hospital therapy section
- Your local gym may even have classes designed for arthritis, heart patients, breast cancer survivors, or senior citizens that would all be helpful for lymphedema and lipedema patients as well.

- The Lipedema Education Group is working to share lipedema, lymphedema and Dercum's disease care guidelines for medical professionals, people with these conditions and their caregivers. Their website is adding information regularly.

QR Link to Lipedema Education Group Website.

- YMCA.org to find local classes for all fitness levels

QR Link to YMCA.org website.

Supply List with Links

If you'd like links to some items on my Aqua therapy supply list, I am keeping a living list, updated on LegsLikeMine.com, on the page below.

I may find other goodies that prove to be helpful and will add them to my online list as I discover them.

Just scan the QR code and it'll take you there!

QR Link to LegsLikeMine's "Living" Aqua therapy Supplies List.

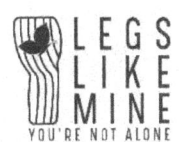

Search Terms and Hashtags that might be helpful:

If you're looking for more information online, using places like YouTube, Instagram, Facebook, Twitter, TikTok, or Google, here's a good starter list of search terms that I used in researching for this book, and might be helpful for you:

Aqua Exercise	Hydrotherapy	Pool exercise
Aqua Fit	Hydropathy	Pool fitness
Aqua Flow	Lipedema Exercise	Swimming
Aqua Lymphatic Therapy	Lymphedema Exercise	Water Aerobics
Aqua Jogging	Plus Swim	Water Cure
Aqua Stretch	Pool exercise	Water Cycling
Aqua therapy	Pool fitness	Water Exercise
AquaFit XXL	Swimming	Water Pedometers
Aquathon	Water Aerobics	Water Treadmill
Fluid Running	Hydrotherapy	Water Walking
LegsLikeMine	Hydropathy	Water Zumba
	Plus Size Swim	

Behind the Scenes Fun

My daughter, Morgan helping me with pre-shoot makeup for LegsLikeMine.com and some of the images in this book.

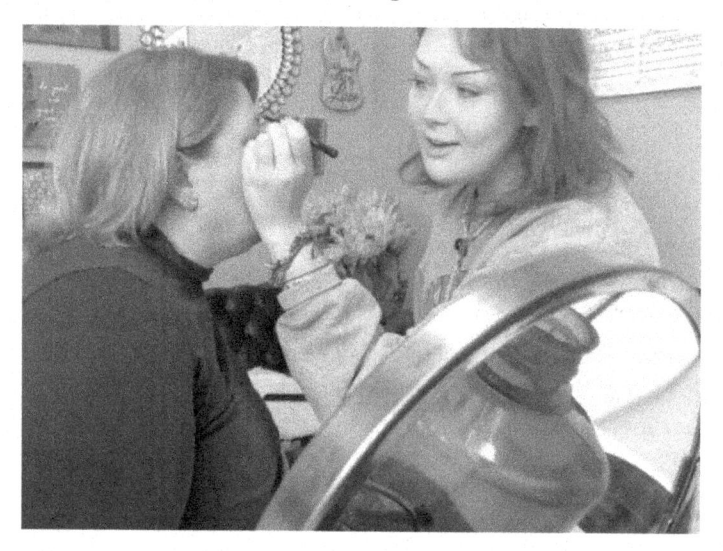

My husband (Rob O'Hara) spent hours in January, February and March fighting the winter weather to help me make this book for you!

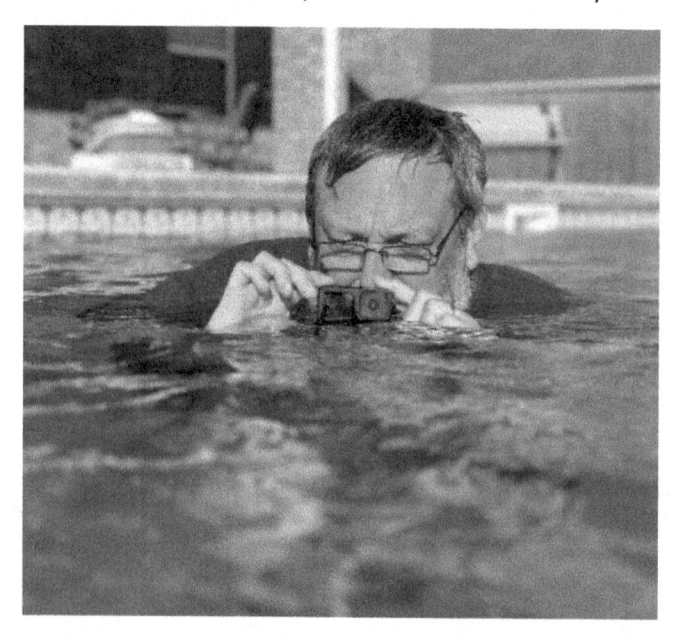

Aqua Therapy for Lipedema and Lymphedema

A behind the scenes look at our portable photo studio action, right in the living room. Our cat even got involved in the picture taking. You'll see more behind the scenes fun on **www.LegsLikeMine.com.**

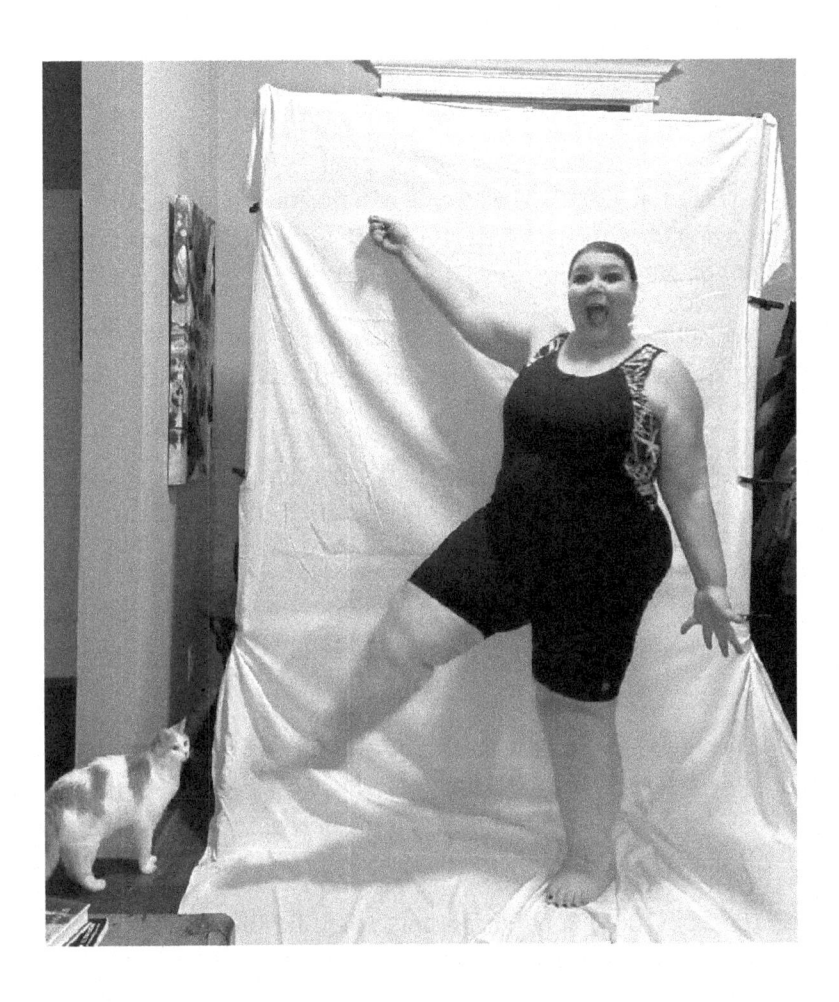

Bibliography

This book would not be possible without the foundation of research that I've been reading for the last two years in preparation for the manuscript writing. Thank you so much to dedicated researchers, medical professionals, and physical trainers for your body of work. You are helping people by sharing what you've learned and teach.

Aquatics

Abou-Dest, A. et al. (2012) "Swimming as a positive moderator of cognitive aging: A cross-sectional study with a multitask approach" Journal of Aging Research.

Alkatan, M., et al (2016). "Improved function and reduced pain after swimming and cycling training in patients with osteoarthritis." The Journal of Rheumatology.

Baines, Susan et al. Aquatic Exercise for Pregnancy: A Resource Book for Midwives and Health and Fitness Professionals. (2010): 48-51.

Birkenfeld et al. (2005) Lipid Mobilization with Physiological Atrial Natriuretic Peptide Concentrations in Humans, The Journal of Clinical Endocrinology & Metabolism, 90(6): 3622–3628. doi.org/10.1210/jc.2004-1953.

Broach, Ellen and McKenney, Alexis. Social Fun and Enjoyment: Viable Outcomes in Aquatics for Individuals with Physical Disabilities. *International Journal of Aquatic Research and Education*: Vol. 6: No. 2, Article 8, 2012. http://scholarworks.bgsu.edu/ijare/vol6/iss2/8.

Bruce E. Becker (2009) Aquatic Therapy: Scientific Foundations and Clinical Rehabilitation Applications, PM&R, 1(9): 859-872. doi.org/10.1016/j.pmrj.2009.05.017.

Bumgardner, Wendy. Verywell Fit.com. Which Pedometers will work underwater? https://www.verywellfit.com/underwater-pedometer-3975552. 02-09-2022.

Burger et al. (2019) Effect of aqua-cycling as exercise therapy in the diagnosis of lipedema. Phlebologie, 48(03): 182-186. DOI: 10.1055/a-0839-6346.

Convert Foot of Water (4°C) to millimeter of mercury (0°C). https://www.convertunits.com/from/feet+of+water/to/mmHg.

Dionne, Andree. Aquatic exercise training and lymphedema. The creation and studied benefits of an aquatic gym. How training in water benefits the body. https://lymphoedemaeducation.com.au/wp-content/uploads/2019/09/Aquatic-exercise-training-and-lymphedema.pdf.

Document, C. (2020) "The Diagnosis and treatment of peripheral lymphedema: 2020 consensus document of the International Society of Lymphology," *Lymphology* 53(1), 3-19.
doi: https://doi.org/10.2458/lymph.4649.

Ergin, Gülbin et al. "Effects of Aqua-Lymphatic Therapy on Lower Extremity Lymphedema: A Randomized Controlled Study." *Lymphatic research and biology* 15 3 (2017): 284-291.

Gianesini et al. (2017) A specifically designed aquatic exercise protocol to reduce chronic lower limb edema. Phlebology, 32(9): 594-600. doi: 10.1177/0268355516673539.

Herbst K. L. (2012). Rare adipose disorders (RADs) masquerading as obesity. *Acta pharmacologica Sinica*, *33*(2), 155–172. https://doi.org/10.1038/aps.2011.153.

Johansson, Karin I et al. "Water-Based Exercise for Patients with Chronic Arm Lymphedema: A Randomized Controlled Pilot Trial." *American Journal of Physical Medicine & Rehabilitation* 92 (2013): 312–319.

Kazutaka F. et al. (1998). Thermoregulatory Responses to Low-Intensity Prolonged Swimming in Water at Various Temperatures and Treadmill Walking on Lad. Eur Journal of Physiological Anthropology and Applied Human Science.
https://www.jstage.jst.go.jp/article/jpa/20/3/20_3_199/_pdf.

Lipodem Mode: Sport with lipedema: Aqua Fitness – exercise in water. 17 April 2018. https://www.lipoedemmode.de/en/aqua-fitness/.

Lipoedema Ladies. Water Magic: Get fit and soothe your symptoms with a water workout. https://www.lipoedemaladies.com/sharie-swimming-lipoedema.

Living Well Institute. Lymphedema, Lipedema dn Aquatic Therapy with PYT. https://proyogatherapy.org/lymphedema-lipedema-and-aquatic-therapy-with-pyt/?fbclid=IwAR01Swu6z8cCwQyi08o5B8zMvM69TuwKN64OqWysVwxv2gw9KC95Po_wIDk.

Mason, Maureen. Lymphedema, Lipedema, and Aquatic Therapy with Professional Yoga Therapy. https://integrativelifestylemed.com/lymphedema-lipedema-and-aquatic-therapy-with-pyt/.

McKenzie, Geoff. World Cancer Day: Treating Lymphedema with Hydrotherapy. https://clearcomfort.com/blog/lymphedema-hydrotherapy-treatment/.

Peyow Aqua Pilates. www.aquapilates.net, and on YouTube: https://www.youtube.com/watch?v=lAND_0kSCZ8.

The Journal of Alternative and Complementary Medicine (JACM). "Aquatic exercise training outcomes on functional capacity, quality of life and lower limb lymphedema." 2018 Sep/ Oct;24(9-10):1007-1009. doi: 10.1089/acm.2018.0041. https://www.ncbi.nlm.nih.gov/pubmed/30247973.

Therapy Achievements, LLC. Water Exercise for Lipedema and Lymphedema. https://therapy-a.com/water-exercise-for-lipedema-and-lymphedema/?fbclid=IwAR3T_0DTVJkQGwEpxiHGv8TxIMnPoNd8Kd9wR1Qu5fGKHzRMVdXkF8yK5_c. 4 July 2020.

Tidhar, D, and Katz-Leurer, M. Aqua lymphatic therapy in women who suffer from breast cancer related lymphedema: a randomized controlled study. *Supportive Care in Cancer*, 2010; 18: 383-392. http://link.springer.com/article/10.1007/s00520-009-0669-4.

Tidhar, D. Aqua Lymphatic Therapy – An Alternate Approach to Controlling Lymphedema. LymphLink Article Reprint 2012. https://nebula.wsimg.com/eb56b44b4597e1c61d6f2fd95f299c84?AccessKeyId=B2CB5B1C9C8FEECF595A&disposition=0&alloworigin=1.

Vécseyné, Magdolna, et. al. Effects of Pilates and aqua fitness training on older adults' physical functioning and quality of life. *Biomedical Human Kinetics*, 2013; 5, 22–27. http://www.degruyter.com/view/j/bhk.2013.5.issue-1/bhk-2013-0005/bhk-2013-0005.pdf.

Vein Center. How to Wear and Care for Compression Stockings: All Stockings are Note Equal. https://veinreliever.com/how-to-wear-and-care-for-compression-stockings/.

Wilcock et al. (2006) Physiological Response to Water Immersion. Sports Med, 36, 747–765. doi.org/10.2165/00007256-200636090-00003.

Lipedma

Fat Disorders Resource Society. Lipedema. https://www.fatdisorders.org/lipedema.

Fife, Caroline, Maus, Erik , Carter, Marissa, Lipedema: A frequently Misdiagnosed and Misunderstood Fatty Deposition Syndrome, *Advances in Skin and Wound Care.* Feb 2010;23(2), 81-92. doi:10.1097/01.asw.0000363503.92360.91.

Forner-Cordero, I, Szolnoky,G, Forner-Cordera, A, Kemeny, L. Lipedema:an overview of its clinical manifestations, diagnosis and treatment of the disproportional fatty deposition syndrome-a systematic review, *Clinical Obesity.* 2012;2(3-4):86-95. doi:10.1111/j.1758-8111.2012.00045.x.

Herbst, Karen L et al. "Standard of care for lipedema in the United States." Phlebology vol. 36,10 (2021): 779-796. doi:10.1177/02683555211015887.

Lipedema.com. Lymphedema vs. Lipedema. https://www.lipedema.com/basics-introduction.

175

Lipedema Foundation. Transformative Publications. https://www.lipedema.org/publications.

Ofabamberg. Lipedema and exercise: Is lipedema resistant to exercise? https://www.ofa-bamberg.com/en/knowledge/clinical-picture/lipedema/lipedema-and-sport/?fbclid=IwAR3eEnWlhiDIXRKXoGxaIHKXQjPLqbS5q3NUSrqfX13sAMingsu8xVxV6pQ.

Okhovat JP, Alavi A. Lipedema: A Review of the Literature. *Int J Low Extrem Wounds*. 2015 Sep;14(3):262-7. doi: 10.1177/1534734614554284. Epub 2014 Oct 17.

Rudkin G, Miller T, Lipedema: A Clinical Entity Distinct from Lymphedema. *Plastic and Reconstructive Surgery*. 1994; 94 (6). doi:10.1097/00006534-199411000-00014 http://journals.lww.com/plasreconsurg/Abstract/1994/11000/Lipedema__A_Clinical_Entity_Distinct_from.14.aspx.

Shin BW, Sim Y-J, Jeong HJ, Kim GC. Lipedema, a Rare Disease. Ann Rehabil Med Annals of Rehabilitation Medicine. 2011 Dec; 35(6): 922–927. doi:10.5535/arm.2011.35.6.922 www.ncbi.nlm.nih.gov/pmc/articles/PMC3309375/.

Lymphedema, Fibrosis and Oncology

American Cancer Society. What is Lymphedema? https://www.cancer.org/treatment/treatments-and-side-effects/physical-side-effects/swelling/lymphedema/what-is-lymphedema.html.

Kwan ML, Cohn JC, Armer JM, Stewart BR, Cormier JN. Exercise in patients with lymphedema: a systematic review of the contemporary literature. Journal of Cancer Survivorship. 2011;5(4):320-336. doi:10.1007/s11764-011-0203-9.

The Mayo Clinic. Physical Medicine and Rehabilitation. "Lymphedema: Diagnosis and treatment." Aug 21, 2018. https://www.mayoclinic.org/medical-professionals/physical-medicine-rehabilitation/news/lymphedema-diagnosis-and-treatment/mac-20436554.

Narahari SR, Ryan TJ, Bose KS, Prasanna KS, Aggithaya GM. Integrating modern dermatology and Ayurveda in the treatment of vitiligo and lymphedema in India. International Journal of Dermatology. 2011;50(3):310-334. doi:10.1111/j.1365-4632.2010.04744.x.

Narahari SR, Ryan TJ, and Aggithaya MG. How Does Yoga Work in Lymphedema? J Yoga Phys Ther. 2013; 03 (02):135. doi:10.4172/2157-7595.1000135.

Petrek JA, Pressman PI, Smith RA. Lymphedema: current issues in research and management. CA: A Cancer Journal for Clinicians. 2000;50(5):292-307. doi:10.3322/canjclin.50.5.292.

Rodrick JR, Poage E, Wanchai A, Stewart BR, Cormier JN, Armer JM. Complementary, Alternative, and Other Noncomplete Decongestive Therapy Treatment Methods in the Management of Lymphedema: A Systematic Search and Review. Pm&r. 2014;6(3):250-274. doi:10.1016/j.pmrj.2013.09.008 http://www.pmrjournal.org/article/S1934-1482(13)01082-4/abstract.

Saravu R. Narahari, Madhur Guruprasad Aggithaya, Kodimoole S. Prasanna, and Kuthaje S. Bose. An Integrative Treatment for Lower Limb Lymphedema (Elephantiasis). *The Journal of Alternative and Complementary Medicine.* February 2010, 16(2): 145-149. doi:10.1089/acm.2008.0546 http://online.liebertpub.com/doi/abs/10.1089/acm.2008.0546?journalCode=acm.

Tiwari A, Cheng KS, Button M, et al. Differential Diagnosis, Investigation, and Current Treatment of Lower Limb Lymphedema. Archives of Surgery. 2003; 138 (2): 152-161. doi:10.1001/archsurg.138.2.152.

Wynn TA, Ramalingam TR. Mechanisms of fibrosis: therapeutic translation for fibrotic disease. Nat Med. 2012 Jul 6;18(7):1028-40. doi: 10.1038/nm.2807. PMID: 22772564; PMCID: PMC3405917.

Wynn TA. Cellular and molecular mechanisms of fibrosis. J Pathol. 2008 Jan;214(2):199-210. doi: 10.1002/path.2277. PMID: 18161745; PMCID: PMC2693329.

Other Resources

Dolyna, Lana. Deducting a Swimming Pool: Do You Qualify? + FAQs. 2022 June. Deducting a Swimming Pool in 2023: Do You Qualify? + FAQs (taxsharkinc.com).

The Ehlers-Danlos Society. hEDS Diagnostic Checklist. https://www.ehlers-danlos.com/heds-diagnostic-checklist/.

Internal Revenue Service. Medical and Dental Expenses for use in preparing 2022 returns. Publication 502. 2022 Publication 502 (irs.gov).

Morrison, T. American Classification of Compression Stockings. http://www.tagungsmanagement.org/icc/images/stories/PDF/morrison_american_classification.pdf.

OpenAI. "ChatGPT." Accessed March 15, 2023. https://openai.com/chat-gpt/.

VimVigr. What is mmHg and What Compression Level is Right for You? 5 May 2022. https://vimvigr.com/blogs/our-blog/what-is-mmhg-how-to-choose-compression-socks?gclid=Cj0KCQiAjbagBhD3ARIsANRrqEs-PJjcAOQkruQpT9ExKnljAIPnRjoybe5VXWntdkF4ROb_d4PvEqUaArMtEALw_wcB.

Connect with LegsLikeMine

Visit us Online at: www.LegsLikeMine.com

To read blog posts, see questions about all kinds of lipedema and lymphedema-related topics answered, hear personal stories, and even get product recommendations for women with lipedema and lymphedema.

Join us on social media for more interaction and additional content:

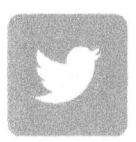

https://www.instagram.com/legs_likemine/?hl=en

https://www.facebook.com/LegsLikeMine/

https://youtube.com/c/LegsLikeMine

https://twitter.com/legs_likemine

https://www.pinterest.com/LegsLikeMine/

Tell us what you think! To share your thoughts, ask a question, submit a product for review, and see what's going on in the lipedema community, please visit: https://LegsLikeMine.com/subscribe/

Susan O'Hara is from Yukon, Oklahoma, and is the founder of LegsLikeMine, LLC. Susan has been affected with lipedema and lymphedema for more than two decades, starting with the birth of her first child in 2001. Her condition progressed slowly through various hormonal changes but flared to a new level with a significantly stressful event that served as the catalyst for seeking surgical treatments.

Like many, Susan went undiagnosed for almost 20 years, suffering pain and slowly losing mobility. Despite diet, exercise, and having two weight-loss surgeries, the condition persisted. After numerous MRIs, knee surgeries, x-rays, and a bout with tendonitis, a technician asked Susan who was treating her lymphedema, and this got her connected to support groups, who actually saw her pictures and suggested she had an advanced stage of lipedema, called Lipo-Lymphedema, where both conditions exist.

Susan's informal, online diagnosis allowed her to begin research, finding specialists and therapists familiar with lipo-lymphedema, who were able to clinically diagnose and provide treatment. Through her research she discovered compression, bandaging wraps and massage techniques to help manage her condition. In 2021, Susan had three Lymph-Sparing Lipectomy surgeries, and incorporated a regular swimming routine into her life to help manage her condition. Throughout her journey, Susan documented everything online on www.LegsLikeMine.com and associated social media platforms, including YouTube.

Her sharing online has opened up opportunities for Susan to do in-person education and speaking events with groups like Girl Scouts, in order to spread awareness of her conditions and get people into treatment earlier, to avoid disease progression. She recently retired from the Federal Aviation Administration, where she just won the Agency's Humanitarian Award for her work with both Lipedema Awareness and Girl Scouts and is dedicating her work now to lipedema education full time.

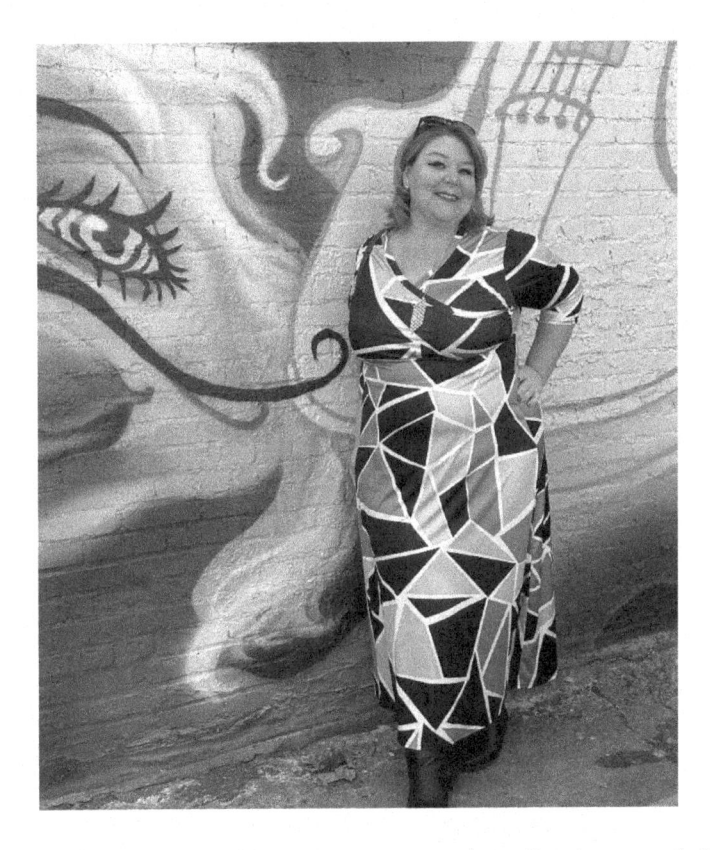

In 2022, Susan was filmed for a documentary about lipedema, and she also created a Girl Scout badge for lipedema awareness.

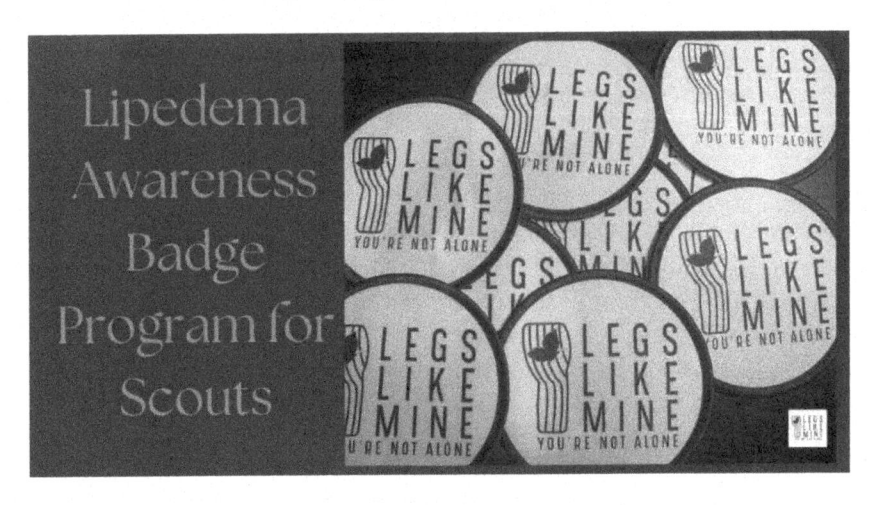

Susan and her mother, who also has the conditions, have struggled for years to find boots, shoes and clothes that fit and help highlight features other than their legs. Susan has dedicated a portion of her social media presence to help others with the condition continue to find and showcase their own beauty and belonging by sharing her fun ideas in fashion in her own, fun, way. She is the author of Jeans on a Beach Day: A Book for the Beautiful Woman Hiding Her Legs (2022), and she is creating a specialty line of footwear for ladies who have lipedema and lymphedema, due out in Winter 2023-24.

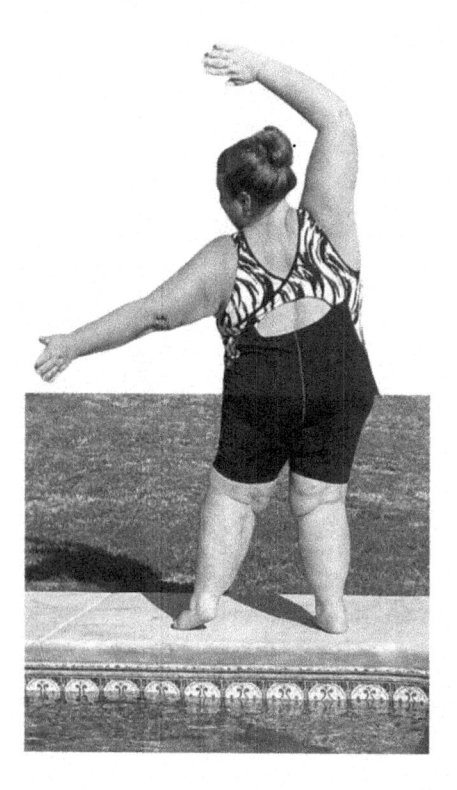

LegsLikeMine is a work of passion and necessity in hopes that it will get products information to people who badly need help and who may not know they have the painful fat conditions called lipedema and lymphedema, or how to manage them.